Do Not Go Gently

Patric Morgan
Copyright © 2012 Patric Morgan
All rights reserved.
ISBN-10: 1480066966
ISBN-13: 978-1480066960

More from Patric Morgan at
www.patricmorgan.co.uk

DEDICATION

This book is dedicated to my wonderful family, who have not only endured a year from hell, but allowed me to write openly and candidly about their experiences.

I would also like to dedicate this book to my wonderful wife Clare and to my close friends who have helped me through the process.

Last, but by no means the least, I'd also like to dedicate this book to my beautiful cat (and writing buddy for many years), who we sadly lost along the way.

I love you all.

"Beautiful. [His] observations as a family member are so insightful that I almost feel part of it." *L Hugglestone*

"…a beautiful writer." *A Morgan*

"It exudes love and warmth." *M Unwin*

"So well written…it shows family relationships in all their beauty." *S Bradley*

"I'm hooked! …..a fantastic writer. I'm in awe and I can't wait to get five minutes to myself to catch up tomorrow." *C Thomas*

"Inspiring and beautiful." *L Oatway*

"Touching and brave." *Boyd Clack*

"A beautiful, moving and personal account." *Dr D Dummett*

"Amazing. I know exactly what you are going through." *Ruth Wignall*

"I've been sitting here reading your blog in tears, but it's a wonderful piece of work." *C Jones*

"Fantastic." *Z Shirley-Smith*

"I read your blog tonight from start to finish in tears and in laughter. I couldn't stop once I'd started. Such an emotive and passionate account and so beautifully written." *A Taylor*

"Fantastic." *L Rae*

"A gifted writer." *S Cross*

"[A] touching blog on a family's dealings with cancer. Moving and gripping, urging the reader not just to read more but to wish the family well as they're welcomed into personal, humorous and character-rich details of the writer's life." *Judges at the 2012 Wales Blog Awards*

"Beautiful and descriptive and such a difficult subject." *K Allen*

"Incredibly moving...you MUST read this wonderfully written blog!" *Ruthie Davies (Winner of 'Best Blog in Wales' and 'Best Writing in a Blog' 2010)*

"More than a worthy winner of 'Best Writing on a Blog'." *A Williams*

CONTENTS

FOREWORD

This story was originally written as an ongoing blog during the summer of 2012. For me, it was my way of dealing with challenging events and emotions.

There are some 'flashbacks' to happier times. These are indicated with ***date***, as these may not manifest themselves in the best way on paper.

For those of you outside of Wales where this story was set, you may come across a few words and/or phrases that are unfamiliar. The first of these, 'cwtch' (pronounced 'cutch') is a Welsh word meaning 'safe', but we now mostly use it to describe a cuddle. One other phrase which pops up in the book a lot is 'pepper pasties'. Although not specific to Wales, they are specific to a baker's shop called the Jolly Baker in our home town. These pasties are very much like corned beef pasties, except that their pastry is a very thin shortcrust pastry and its fillings are a little more peppery than most. They usually sell out by 1pm and the chef there never discloses the recipe to me, no matter how many times I ask him.

Patric Morgan, November 2012

PROLOGUE

Early April 2012 5.30am

Nan had slipped away in the early hours. We were half-expecting it, but even so, it hurt. So we stayed up all night, talking and drinking milky tea. And as daylight broke, we went to the beach to watch the sunrise.

It was a warm morning. As the sky stretched and yawned, Mum, my sister and I huddled over a piping flask of coffee. The sand was cold and a slight breeze whispered in from the darkness. Even though Nan had only died a few hours earlier, Mum couldn't stop talking about Dad. She was so worried about his refusal to visit a doctor.

She sipped her coffee. "Dad and I came here when we were courting back in the late sixties. We were sat on that headland over there. We cwtched for hours and with my head on his chest, I could hear his heart beating. I remember thinking even then, what would I do if it stopped beating?"

Late April 2012

Hidden away in the middle room of the Victorian house in Barry, sat my father. I hadn't been there for weeks. You know how it gets. Work picks you up like some gust of wind and dumps you months down the line. Dad was never the most social of people, yet seeing him sat on the settee, reading the papers and listening to the cricket on a small portable radio seemed poignant. While the house around him buzzed with life and laughter, he'd shut himself away and watched and listened as life carried on around him.

Looking back, I think he knew then that he wasn't very well. Back in 2008, when my sister Mari was diagnosed with cancer in her knee, my Dad lost his voice. We thought it was the shock. But even when Mari came out the other side, Dad's voice never made it. We had lost the voice of our childhood.

But since early 2012, it wasn't just his voice that was causing concern. His breathing had become a real struggle. We could hear him from the other end of the house. My feeling is that he'd now become such an embarrassment, that he didn't want to impose it on the family. When we'd ask how he was coping with his breathing, he'd act surprised.

"There's nothing wrong with my breathing!" he'd say, like a child lying about breaking a parent's precious statue.

But eventually, he started avoiding the questions by retiring to the sitting room and making himself a little haven. When I saw him there, he seemed to have shrunk into the settee. He wasn't the giant of a man who had scooped me up in his arms and thrown me up into the air as a kid, only to catch me again and give me one of those big hugs that only dads give.

May 2012

It was my brother Dan who had finally seemed to twist Dad's arm and get him to the doctor. They had no records of him there - the last time he'd seen a doctor was back in the late fifties. He finally got seen to and they sent him for tests. I'm not sure of the exact series of events but I do know that both him and my mother had planned to head down to West Wales on his birthday. West Wales to my dad is his solace. About ten years ago, when he'd been made redundant, he'd planned to buy himself a static caravan where he could escape the intensity of family life. My mum's family is a big one and he'd often hide himself away when they arrived. They loved him all the same. But West Wales was where he grew up and where he'd sit on the beach at Saundersfoot and picture himself with the family that we no longer there.

So West Wales was where they were heading for his birthday until he had a letter from the hospital informing him that he had an appointment the same day. Dad, wanting to head west to avoid seeing the doctor, was furious. My mum, wanting my dad to face what could be going on, was also furious. They called the hospital to rearrange. Later that day, they sat in the car, eating a bag of chips outside a church in Saundersfoot. It was raining and there was a funeral going on.

"This is heaven. Bliss." said Dad.

Mum rolled her eyes in disbelief.

1. RAINY DAYS AND PEPPER PASTIES

Thursday 14th June 2012

I wasn't expecting the phone call.

I was on 'standby' to pick Dad up from the hospital if the results were bad, but we were pretty confident that the doctors would send him home and that would be that. But the instant that I saw that Mum was calling, I knew.

"Hello?"

"Hi. Can you come pick us up please?"

"It's bad isn't it?"

"Yes."

"What is it?"

"I'll tell you when you get here."

"Tell me now. It's fine. I don't want things going through my head when I'm driving. I'd rather know."

I knew that whatever Mum threw at me next, I had to act calm and cool.

"It's cancer of the larynx."

I sucked in a big breath.

"Ok. I'll be there in ten minutes."

"Thanks."

***

I was stood alone in the kitchen looking at the floor. I felt like I'd just been smashed over the back of the head with one of the flagstones. There was a flutter of panic rising up inside me. The same sort of panic that'd overwhelmed me four years earlier when I had a similar phone call from Mum about my 14 year old sister Mari. I was teaching that day, and ran limp-legged through Pontypool Park to the train station in the rain to get home. It was raining today too. I looked out through the rain-rippled kitchen window into the garden.

Where had summer gone?

I arrived at the hospital but had another phone call to say that Dad was driving himself home. I think he wanted to get as far away from the hospital as quickly as he could. I caught sight of their car leaving the hospital and went chasing after it.

I could make out the shape of Dad's head driving as we headed out of the city. I wondered what was going through it and felt like some kind of over-protective outrider as I tried to shield him from other drivers around him. My phone rang on my hands-free.

"Hello?"

"Hi. It's Danielle. How did it go?" (Danielle has been a very good friend of mine for the last 20 years)

"Not well. It's cancer of the larynx." With that, my voicebox broke and I couldn't speak.

"Oh no. Oh love. I don't know what to say. I'm so sorry."

I still couldn't speak. I couldn't stop crying. We eventually spoke about what happened next. We spoke about smoking and the shit it causes. We spoke about what Mari my sister had been through. And before I knew it, I was back at my parents' house.

I pulled up and could see that Mum was already in the house. Dad was getting out of the car alone. My tears were still coming. I didn't dare rub my eyes and make them all red. I had to pretend that I was on the phone while I sucked them all back in. I finally got out of the car to find him waiting for me. He still looked the same. For some reason, I expected him to look ill.

For a few moments, it was just the two of us hugging.

"You hungry?" I asked.

"I wasn't but I am now."

"Pepper pasty?"

"Aye. Loads of them. And some custard slices too. Let's stuff our fucking faces." said Dad.

2 A PAIR OF CRUTCHES

Thursday 14th June 2012

"How many pasties have you had?" asked Dylan.

"Erm… this is my fourth." I replied as I sank my teeth into another hot pasty.

"Jesus. No wonder you're 15 stone."

"Oi. My body's a temple." I said.

"Aye. A Temple of Doom." came Dylan, stirring a sugar into his tea.

Dylan, my youngest brother seemed unfazed at the news. He was still talking about the latest song he'd written and wanted me to promote. Dad brought us all a cup of tea to the dining table. This was the table where life's problems got solved. It had seen us through decades of Christmas dinners, endless Saturday night fry-ups, and summer parties. It had seen me through school homework and my degree. It was also the place where Beti, my other younger sister (only by a year or so) announced to the family that she was pregnant at the age of 15. I hugged Dad that night. I found him crying in the sitting room where he'd now taken up camp nearly twenty years later. He told me that I was his 'rock'.

So here we were again, at the table, plotting our next adventure. This is how we got our heads around things. In this case, it was pasties and cakes.

I left the house later that day with a heavy heart. Despite all the banter and laughter, I knew that there were some tough times ahead. It wasn't going to be pretty.

Saturday 23rd June 2012

A week later, we hadn't heard anything from the hospital. I had a school reunion at a local pub planned on the Saturday, which I was thinking about pulling out of but I'm glad I went. Even though it was twenty years since I last saw my school friends, everyone was the same. Fergus, one of my good friends was still putting his foot in it.

"So you're a grandmother now then Emma?"

"Am I?" replied Emma, spluttering her drink all down her top.

"Yes. I'd read somewhere that your daughter...you got a daughter right?"

"Yes."

"I'd read that she'd had a kid."

"Not that I know of." she said, mopping down her blouse.

"Oh."

There was a tumbleweed moment until someone piped up:

"Still charming the ladies then Ferg?"

Sat in the corner was my friend Rich. He was very quiet, not the Rich I knew from school. Next to him were two crutches, propped up against the wall.

"Who's on crutches?"

My mate Matt turned to me.

"Rich. He's got MS." That shut me up for a few minutes.

Later on, I watched Rich struggle to get to the gents. It was heart-breaking. I got talking to him later and he came out his shell a little.

The next day, he posted on Facebook about what a good night he'd had and how it was the first time he had socialised for two years, how it had boosted his confidence. It made me realise that Dad was going to need his confidence propped up over the next few months. I was going to have to be a crutch to lean on. A rock.

Later that day, I had a call from Mum.

"Can you come to the hospital with us on Monday please? We've got to see the doctors to see what happens next."

3 PEGS AND MAGIC COINS

Monday 25th June 2012

I'd got stuck in the notorious Cardiff rush-hour traffic and arrived at the hospital an hour later than I'd wanted. The rest of my family were in 'the meeting' so I had no way of finding out where they were until someone happened to look at their phone.

I eventually found them in a small meeting room. Dad was sat opposite an empty chair. Mum was sat next to him and over in the corner were my two sisters, Beti and Mari. I had to squeeze myself into the corner behind Dad so that I was stood behind him. It was probably just as well as I didn't want to see the worry on his face.

A surgeon-type person walked in, introduced himself and sat in the empty seat. He was very routine. He rattled off questions and ticked some boxes. My younger sister Mari laughed at every question and the surgeon looked at her every time she did, half-expecting her to explain what she was laughing at. She wasn't finding it funny. She had 'laughed' when she had been told that she had cancer at the age of 14. It was nerves.

"Do you mind if I look down your throat?" asked the surgeon. Mari laughed.

"Yes." said Dad.

"You do mind?"

"Yes I do. I had it done a few weeks back and it was hell. You saw what was there and you even took photos. Look at them. I'm not having another tube shoved down my throat."

I was taken aback at Dad's assertiveness. I'd never seen it before. Not ever.

The surgeon was stuck for words too. He chewed on his pen and thought for a while before moving on to the next question.

After he'd gone, a lovely lady came in who told us what the plan was likely to be. Dad was told that he'd have to have a PEG fitted - a tube that he could feed himself directly into his stomach with, should the radiotherapy prove too harsh on his throat. Dad's stomach had always been important to him, and he seemed to accept it with some reluctance. Besides, putting stuff straight into one's belly takes away the pleasure of eating. Those pepper pasties weren't going to taste the same.

The lady left and Dad stood up, pacing back and forth.

He had nowhere to go.

"Can't wait to get out of this bloody place." he muttered. I mumbled something about being patient and Dad said that he had no choice but to be a patient. We all laughed a nervous laugh.

The last consultant-type person left and we were finally free to go, albeit for one last X-ray. We headed down to A&E where we passed an old woman we'd known from church on a stretcher in a corridor. We were all a bit surprised to see each other in a hospital setting - she didn't look safe without the sanctuary of a church around her. She'd also always had big bulging eyes, and the sight of us coming around the corner made it look as if she'd still had a thermometer stuck up her arse.

******April 1974******

"What time do you start work?"

Dad mumbled some kind of reply into his pillow. He hadn't slept well, worrying about the first day in his new job.

"What time are you working?" Mum asked again. Dad raised his head, bleary-eyed and ruffle haired.

"What? What are you on about?" he asked.

Mum sighed. "What time are you starting work? I thought it was 8 and it's quarter to now..."

"Shit!"

Mum hadn't had time to finish her sentence before Dad was scrambling out of bed. The bedroom was small and Dad was trapped in the corner of the bed, which was up against the wall. He hopped over her, flashing a pair of dangling bollocks in Mum's face, before flinging open the bedroom door and dashing downstairs.

"Good luck." mumbled Mum as she rolled back over to rest, cradling the baby within her.

******

Sunday 1st July 2012

In many ways, Sunday lunch with the parents seemed like the Last Supper. It would be the last time for a while that we could all sit around the family table without drugs and feeding tubes to think about. Tomorrow he'd be in hospital having the PEG fitted.

I wasn't sure whether I was the only one feeling nervous but Dad was quieter than normal. He was also giving more hugs than usual. Mari was drifting around the house, cursing the drunken ramble she'd given her boyfriend the night before. I think she was getting nervous too.

"Make my coin disappear again." said Harri. Dan's 6 year old boy always had a smile on his face. Harri and I were sat on the settee in the living room together.

Harri was always fascinated when I used to use sleight of hand to make his coins disappear and reappear behind his ear. Only a few weeks ago, when everything was ok, we were at the bottom of the staircase. I made his coin disappear as usual and then told him that I'd make it reappear at the top of the stairs. As he looked up the stairs and then back at me, I'd thrown the coin up the stairs without him seeing. I then told him that he'd find his coin at the top.

He was amazed when he found his coin there.

"Make my coin appear at the top of the stairs again." he demanded. As we were on the settee in the living room, there was no way I could make the coin reappear at the top of the stairs this time.

It seemed my magic could only stretch so far.

I wondered at the beauty of his innocence as I looked at him smiling at me. I felt sorry that one day, he'd grow up and realise the ugly truth that I was just having him on; that it was all just a trick.

'Enjoy it.' I thought to myself. 'It won't be long before you'll look back on this and wish you were still here.'

"It was my birthday last week." he said changing the subject.

I'd forgotten. Again.

"Was it?"

"Yes. I had a party. Why didn't you come?"

"Erm...I was working sorry. Did you have nice things?" I said.

"Yes. You'll come to my next one though, right?"

"Of course. Let me know when it is. I'm rubbish at remembering things." Clare, my wife, who was sat on the other settee, shook her head and rolled her eyes, smiling.

I leaned back on the settee and reached into my pocket. I scrunched up the tenner that was in there and held onto it tightly for a few minutes.

"Harri - you've got something...something behind your ear..."

Then I 'pulled out' the tenner from behind his ear.

"WOW!!!" he squealed, before running out to the kitchen to tell Dan.

But Dad noticed that I wasn't smiling. I was still thinking about tomorrow.

"You ok?" he asked.

I sat upright.

"Yeah. Totally fine."

I realised that I had to up my act as Master of Illusion.

4 ANDY MURRAY AND THE GARLIC BURP

Monday 2nd July 2012

"Ward West 2." announced Mum, putting the phone back on its receiver and sighing.

My mug of tea had long gone cold and Serena Williams had just won another game at Wimbledon. It was sunny there. Why was it still raining here?

We trooped out to the car - Dad, Mum, Mari and I. We laughed as we stopped the car at a zebra crossing for a three-legged dog. We'd joked about how he must have learned his lesson last time he tried to cross the road, now only having three legs. And then it went quiet. Out of the corner of my eye, I could see Dad's hand clutching a piece of paper. In the rear view mirror, I looked to see if Mum and Mari were on their phones as they were silent too. But they were both gazing out of the windows, watching the low clouds dragging their feet across the fields.

The first thing that hit us on the ward was the smell. That old man, pissy kind of smell. Flanking either side of the ward were old men with wonky faces. There was one man with one leg. There was a Chinese-looking man who was watching tennis on a telly no bigger than a shoe box. Dad's bed was right down the end. The curtains had been pulled around the very last bed in the line and as we laid out Dad's bag, we could hear the conversation next to us.

"I'm not a professional. Just a good amateur."

said the male nurse. The curtains flung open. The guy lying on the bed had made himself quite at home. He was resting there on his side, in his jeans, propping his head up on his arm. His portable radio was blasting out Subterranean Homesick Blues, and Mum pointed out that Dad would be right at home.

Feeling awkward, we headed to the 'Day Room'. There were two settees and a woman sat there watching tennis. Bloody tennis.

"I just love Andy Murray." she said to me as I dropped my arse on the sofa with a book about Scott Joplin. She was a well-spoken woman of about 60 years of age.

"Yeah?"

"Oh yes." She bit into a biscuit and smiled at the TV.

"He's got a very small head hasn't he?" I said.

The lady thought for a moment.

"It's because he's very long." she replied.

"Yes. I guess so. If he is very tall, I guess his head would seem further away to us normal people. It's called perspective isn't it?"

The woman continued to eat her biscuit.

4pm came and it was chucking out time. We'd only been seen by a staff nurse but we could tell that Dad was feeling awkward for us. So we headed home in the rain.

Tuesday 3rd July 2012

I had a text from Dad around midday to say that he'd had the PEG fitted, that he was feeling fine and that he'd be having some food later on that day.

I picked up Mum and Mari at half five and once again, we headed out into the rain. The journey to the hospital was uneventful, save for a very large belch courtesy of Mum who was sat next to me. I'd had the blowers on hot to clear the windscreen and the burp hit me like a huge, hot bubble of garlic. Mari, who was sat in the back with her i-Pod on, and who wasn't aware that Mum had burped, piped up:

"What the hell is that smell? It's disgusting!"

"Sorry - that was me." said Mum.

We all wound down our windows and I put the blowers on full blast again. The air was thick with garlic and it took a good few minutes to clear the car of it.

We arrived on the ward. Dad seemed to be the only guy sat up in bed and we spotted his happy-looking head down the bottom of the ward. The place seemed a lot cleaner this time round and we grabbed our seats and dotted them around his bed. The old guy in the bed next to us was tucked up to his chin, eyes closed and looked in some kind of discomfort.

"So it all went ok then?"

"Aye." said Dad, tucking into a Freddo bar that Mum had brought in. "I thought I was going to have a general anaesthetic but all they did was sedate me and cram my gob full of instruments." He seemed pretty calm about it all. I told him that he'd done well.

"Oh no." said Mum, clutching her mouth with her hands. Before she could stop herself, she'd managed to muffle another monster garlic burp.

We all groaned in dismay.

Dad had been smiling until the burp slapped him in the face.

"Eurgh." Even from the other side of the bed, we could taste it.

"Right. I'll get you back for that." said Dad, lifting his blanket and pretending to 'lift a cheek'.

What we hadn't noticed was that three female nurses had pulled the curtain around the old guy in the bed next to us.

"Jesus." said Mum, clutching her nose. "You dirty bastard!" Dad looked shocked, as he hadn't actually done anything.

Then the sweet-smelling aroma of warm shit hit the rest of us over the other side of the bed.

"Pwoar. Dad!!" bawled Mari, covering her face.

"Christ. That smells like baby shit. What the hell have you been eating?" I said, making my point rather loudly.

"Sshhhh..." said Dad. "It's the guy next door. He's having his nappy changed."

We all turned to see the curtains of the bed next to us being opened and the three nurses stepping out. One of them was carrying what looked like a bag of chips in a plastic bag.

There was an awkward silence.

"Erm...Andy Murray won." said Mum, not knowing what to say.

I looked at the old guy next to us who'd just had his bed bath. His eyes were still closed but he now had a smile on his face.

'The old pervert. He's not ill.' I thought to myself.

We were there for a good two hours and visitors were starting to leave. Some of the older guys were bedding down for the night.

"Aw." said Mum. "Look at him over there."

We all looked to see an old guy curling up in a ball and pulling his blankets up to his chin. "He looks cosy."

"That's Des." announced Dad. He was still eating.

"Oo. Check you out. You've become a new man since you've been ill. Before now, you'd never speak to anyone and now here you are on first name terms with everyone on the ward."

"No." said Dad, popping a macaroon into his mouth. "It says his name above the bed."

5 JIM AND THE PYJAMAS

Wednesday 4th July 2012

Dad wasn't happy.

"The doctor said I could come home today until that witch of a dietician turned up and overruled him. Fucker."

Dad was tucking into his KitKat and Mum was sat neatly at his bedside. I'd had a stressful day with work but this was a chance for me to relax somewhat.

In the bed next to us was the guy who'd had his nappy changed yesterday. He was asleep, still tucked up tight like some kind of mummy. A younger man was sat on a chair at his bedside, simply leaning forward and looking at him. I presume it was his son. The son looked about 40 or so. He had a wispy moustache, a grey cardigan and a constant smile. He'd sit there for the next two hours on his own, holding his dad's hand, rolling his thumb over his dad's fingers and occasionally looking around the ward for something to do.

I sat there for a while and imagined what sort of things they'd got up to over the years - long, hot summer days to the beach, autumn drives out to North Wales perhaps. I thought about the day that the dad had held his son in his hands for the first time; the long nights he probably had to endure over the next few years, and the long lonely shifts that he must have put in to look after his family.

Directly opposite my Dad was Jim. Jim

was an older man with large glasses on, probably mid-seventies. He looked like something from the 1950s. Yesterday he'd sat there looking angry but said nothing. Today was the same. He'd have found it hard to say anything as he had an oxygen mask strapped to his face. Oxygen was pouring from either side of the mask. He looked like some kind of dragon, seething with rage. It was only when a nurse walked past that he finally pulled off the mask and said something.

"Excuse me!"

His huge voice boomed down the ward, bouncing off the walls and stirring all the sleeping souls in their beds.

"When can I take this bloody thing off? I've had it on now for a bloody hour. I'm only supposed to have it on for twenty bloody minutes."

The nurse headed over and switched the machine off. Jim repeated what he'd just said but louder, just to make sure she'd heard, and presumably the doctors on the ward next door.

"I've had it on now for a bloody hour. I'm only supposed to have it on for twenty bloody minutes."

The nurse quickly packed the machine away and whisked it back up the ward. Jim was itching for a fight. His fingers dug into his bed and his feet twitched in their bed socks. It was probably just as well that his daughter came in when she did.

"I've just been to Matalan to get you some more pyjamas." she said, reaching into a plastic bag.

Jim waved his arms around.

"I don't want any more bloody pyjamas. I've got loads of the bloody things." he bellowed in his grey, chapel-stone voice. "I don't bloody want them!"

We all looked at each other and stifled our smiles.

"He sounds like Hugh Griffith." said Dad. Jim's daughter had obviously tried to give him something else.

"I don't want your bloody 50p! I don't need anything. What's 50p going to bloody buy me? I can't even get out of this bloody bed to spend bloody 50p." Jim was like a volcano, who'd been waiting for days to erupt. Even the young guy looking at his dad in the bed next to us gave us a knowing look.

Jim carried on with his tirade. Within a few minutes, the entire ward knew that he'd gotten sore ears from the oxygen mask but that he had eaten his custard that had been served for his dessert.

A few whoops came from the Day Room at the end of the ward.

"Oh no. I'm missing the Andy Murray match again." said Mum.

Then there came a few groans. The game had been rained off.

Mari appeared at the door. She'd been out in Cardiff with a friend and had popped in on the way back. Jim was still spouting off and Mari took her seat to be entertained by him.

Dad was still moaning about not being let home. Worse still, they'd told him that he wasn't having lasagna for tea. He'd been looking forward to it all day. What he got was a bowl of corned beef hash instead. I could tell that Dad wasn't going to find this whole thing easy unless it all went to plan.

Mum tried to soothe the situation by pointing out a slipper that was lying abandoned underneath the curtains that had been drawn around a bed opposite. Mum found small things funny.

"Ha - look at that one slipper!" she pointed out.

Dad reminded her that the guy only had one leg and therefore only needed one slipper.

I shook my head. "You're always putting your foot in it." I said without thinking, which probably wasn't the wisest thing to say.

I made a right arse of myself on the way out of the hospital too. I was explaining to Mari what Jim had been like before she arrived. I did what I thought was a very good impersonation of him.

"Bloody pyjamas! Bloody custard!" I bellowed, throwing my arms around, before realising that the woman walking directly in front of us was his daughter. The toes in my shoes curled with embarrassment and I got in the car as quickly as I could.

Later on, after I'd dropped Mum and Mari home, and was heading back home in the car on my own, I switched on the CD player. The evening sun had just come out for the first time in weeks and I fancied some kind of music. The last CD I'd listened to in the car was a Christmas Carols CD and my immediate reaction was to turn it off and put on something else instead.

But as I headed down through the sun-dappled country lanes, this spiritual music seemed oddly appropriate. It reminded me of Christmas Day, only seven months ago, when Clare and I had headed down to Barry to see the family with the same CD on. Back then, the earth did stand hard as iron and the streams along the roadside did stand like stone. But there was warmth to be found at the end of our journey at my parents' house.

There was some warmth from the evening

sun too as I headed home. I hoped that this was maybe the start of some better times. Little was I to know.

6 BULLY BEEF AND THE SLUDGE GULPER

Thursday 5th July 2012

Dad and his small bag were already sat on the bench outside the main entrance of the hospital when I pulled up in the car. He had his face to the sun that had made another rare appearance and he seemed to be enjoying his first fresh air for days.

He seemed like an excited little dog all the way home in the car.

"This is lush." he kept saying. With the windows wound down, the car ambled its way through the countryside towards home. We spotted an airship high above the yellow fields and reminisced about how we'd see them above the street I grew up in as a kid.

Mum had already brought the settee up from the far end of the room up to the coal fire, which she'd just lit when we arrived at the house. Even though it was July, it had been a wet month and she'd had the fire going for the last few days.

"I've just had a toof out." she explained. She stood in front of the mirror that sat on the mantelpiece, opened her mouth and peered in. What she was expecting to see, I don't know but she was keen to point out that she had been 'under the knife' too, albeit at the dentist.

"Old Bully Beef is dead." she announced, mouth still wide open.

"Good God." said Dad. "How old was she?"

"Seventy odd."

I had no idea who they were talking about

but my guess was that they didn't call her that to her face. I headed out to the kitchen where a few saucepans sat bubbling away underneath the cooker hood light. The windows had steamed up and there was a heady smell of meat cooking. Mum had obviously thought this through. I could hear Dad, who was sat right up against the fire.

"This is lush." he kept saying. Then I heard him saying to Mum that he was going to be eating tea like a 'sludge-gulper'.

"That's a marvellous word." I heard him say. "Sludge-gulper." he said to himself rather proudly.

******November 5th 1979******

Dad was on one of his toot'l'ten shifts and Mum had decided to paint the living room windowsills with a tin of gloss paint she'd found under the kitchen sink. She'd started the job at lunchtime but it was already getting dark by half three. Eager to see any early fireworks being let off, my sister Beti and I sat in the front window, waiting for the dark. In our attempts to look down the street, we'd pushed our little hands into the now jelly-like paint and pushed it all the way up to the window in one big smudge. It ruined Mum's paintwork and stayed there until we left ten years later.

******

Friday 6th July 2012
8.15am

That was the time that Dad was waiting for on the oven clock before we had to leave for a kidney function test. The test would determine the levels of chemo he'd get over the next few weeks and it involved injecting him with some substance, and then being subject to hourly blood tests over the course of the morning.

Dad was leaning over to look at the oven clock. It seemed as if he was squeezing out the last few minutes of being at home. Finally the clock silently announced that it was time to move.

"Ok. Let's go." said Dad.

It was a fresh morning and I could smell the beach some two miles away as we headed down the garden path. Heavy rain had been forecast for later in the day. On the way in, Dad told us about Monty the Spider, who lived in the wing mirror of Dad's car. Monty was probably having a whale of a time in Dad's car which lay dormant outside the house.

We arrived at the hospital in good time and found our way to a tiny little room. Dad was asked to head to another room so I escorted him there. The woman opened the door to another small room, where perched on a podium in the middle of the floor was what looked like an electric chair. It probably felt that way for Dad too. He hated needles.

What happened next made for uncomfortable viewing. It was also the first time that Dad had received any kind of treatment in front of me. I could tell that he was trying to be brave but his feet kept tapping on the floor and he kept looking around the room, as if for an escape.

The woman was very friendly. I was Dad's corner-man once again and I kept trying to distract him so that he'd look over to me and not at the needle that was about to go in his arm.

"Ok. Look over to the corner of the room now." said the nurse.

He didn't of course. Instead, he scrunched his face up into a ball and looked at the ceiling.

"There. All done." said the nurse, clamping some tissue down on his arm. She gave us some instructions about coming back in two, three, and four hours.

We decided to drive out to a nearby park for an hour or so. The rain clouds were sat smothering the hills in the distance so we headed in to the café that sat on the lakeside. They were still opening when we got there but it meant that at least the coffee was fresh. Dad ordered a chocolate muffin while Mari took a slice of Victoria sponge. My breakfast was a custard slice that stuck to my fingers but it tasted divine. Once we'd eaten, we stood against the railings overlooking the lake for a while. In the distance, we could see the grey rain clouds swallowing up whole mountains.

We visited the hospital three more times that morning, on the hour, every hour. As Dad and I walked back to the car to head home, he told me that he wanted to fight this thing hard.

"I really appreciate you helping out today. I want to try and keep doing things for myself as long as I can though. I'm not going to sit around feeling sorry for myself."

I thought that was a good attitude to have. I was also pleased as we passed a shrivelled up lady who was sat smoking on a stone wall outside the hospital.

"That's disgusting." he said. "All those people in there trying to make us better and she's out here having a fag. That is an insult."

I took them home when all was done. The kettle was the first thing to go on, followed by the telly and a few lamps. The rain had returned but at

Wimbledon at least, the sun was still shining. Mum dragged the settees around the telly and Dad lit the fire. With piping hot mugs of tea in their hands, they were settled and ready to see if Andy Murray could get to his first Wimbledon final.

"This is lush." said Dad.

'Bloody Andy Murray.' I thought.

7 WILLOW THE WISP AND THE MAGIC ROUNDABOUT

Monday 9th July 2012

We'd all had a weekend off visiting hospitals. I'd managed to get some rest but with it came time to dwell on things. Andy Murray got through to the Wimbledon final alright, but soon went from being British hopeful to plucky Scottish loser.

I don't normally suffer from Monday morning blues as I work from home. And as a writer and publisher, I very much enjoy my work. It is hard. I work alone and have no-one to really speak to in the day. And I have to make myself work as no-one else is going to do it for me.

I spent the morning putting some pages of my latest magazine together so that I'd feel like I'd achieved something with my day. Then I hopped into the car to see an advertiser who was late with their copy. It was while I was driving that my phone rang. I pulled over and answered. It was Mum.

"Hiya. I was wondering if you were around today?"

"I can be. Why?"

"He's had a call from the doctor and he wants to see him today."

"But he's got an appointment tomorrow with the consultant."

"I know. But they still want to see him today." sighed Mum.

My first instinct was to wonder why they couldn't take themselves but when I heard Mum sighing, it dawned on me that this could be more bad news. My stomach knotted.

"Yeah. Course. I'll head on down."

The same old questions started flooding my head: 'What have they found?' 'How long has he got left?'

Our journey to the doctors was made in silence. The waiting room was empty and Boney M were playing on the radio. We were the only people there but we were still made to wait. Then we were called in.

"Ah. How are you?" said the doctor eagerly. He was a small wisp of a man with round spectacles and a tweed jacket on.

"I'm fine." said Dad.

"Good." The doctor looked down at his notes on his desk. "So...erm...you've been to hospital? And what did they say?"

"I've got cancer of the larynx."

"I see. And have they told you what they are going to do about it?"

"Yes. Chemo and radiotherapy."

"Ah. I see..." The doctor tapped a few notes onto his computer. Dad looked at Mum with a slight smirk on his face. The doctor didn't know anything about anything.

"And, this may sound a stupid question," he continued, "but do you have the support of your family?"

My Mum looked at me, stood arms folded in the corner of the room. Dad didn't even have to answer.

"I said it was a stupid question." said the doctor. "Ok. Well. Thank you for coming." he said, reaching out to shake Dad's hand.

And with that, we filed out the door and

back into the car. We all sat there for a second, still in silence before I eventually started the car with a huge sigh and turned the car around for home.

Tuesday 10th July 2012

I arrived at the hospital a little early but Dad's car was already there. We were there to see the consultant. We'd last seen her when she'd laid out the plans for the next few months. Today was about firming up those details and signing the consent form to begin chemo. But Mum was worried. She was convinced that there was something they weren't telling us.

On the way to the hospital, I'd pulled up at a roundabout to see a young Chinese learner driver coming around very slowly. I could see his instructor telling him to come off at my exit but the kid panicked and headed back around the roundabout. I sat waiting for other traffic and before I knew it, the kid had come around again. His instructor pointed once again to my exit and once again, the kid panicked and headed around the roundabout. Rather amused, I sat there and waited to see if he would turn off. As he came around again, the instructor, now looking rather pissed off, pointed decisively at the exit. The kid, still gripping the wheel with fear, ignored the instructor and went around for a third time.

It seemed he couldn't get off the ride he'd set out on. I felt the same.

At the hospital, we were kept waiting once again. Mum was puffing out her cheeks and picking at her nails. Dad was picking up on Mum's nerves. They called him to be weighed. They seemed to do that wherever he went.

They finally called us in and once again, it was a case of squeezing us all in a tiny room. A nurse helped us drag in some chairs and I wedged myself in the corner near a tiny asthmatic window. We waited some more.

"I used to be such an optimist." said Mum, looking down at her fingers. "When I was younger, I brought you all up telling you how wonderful life was going to be. I told you all the positive things. And it doesn't work that way at all. Life is hard. Life is shit sometimes. I haven't even had time to get over our Mam going."

I felt a surge of love for my mum. A small woman, but one who'd done a wonderful job in bringing up five kids and giving us all a wonderful childhood. But things had hit her hard over the last few months. It didn't seem fair. She'd done nothing wrong.

She looked up at Dad who was sat there, leaning way back in his chair. I watched as her eyes stroked him. She clearly still felt a lot of love for him, as she did when she was a teenager. But then she spoke.

"What the hell you got in your pocket? You look like a friggin' packhorse." she said.

Dad jumped up and adjusted his jeans, which had gathered around his crotch to give him one almighty 'mound'. That broke the ice for a second but we quickly slipped back into a quiet, fretful silence.

After twenty minutes or so, the doctor came in. She was a pretty lady, and she neatly sat on the seat in front of Dad with a smile. Behind her came another lady, slightly older and she sat on the couch which was the only space available to sit.

"How are you?" asked the doctor.

Dad nodded. He couldn't speak.

"You all ready?"

Dad nodded again, lips pursed tight. He looked like he was going to burst into tears.

The older lady leaned over to Dad and gripped his arm.

"What's the matter? You expecting us to tell you something different?"

Dad finally spoke, his voice breaking.

"Yes. We were. I'm sorry. I'm nervous."

"Well it's ok. We're not going to tell you anything different." She rubbed his arm.

The doctor went through what we'd been through a few weeks earlier. She talked us through the procedure. Two drugs and five nights in hospital starting tomorrow. Side effects would include sickness, diarrhoea, tiredness, and susceptibility to infection. Mari's eyes were glazed over. I knew she was back in 2008, in her hospital bed. She knew what Dad was about to go through.

The doctor got Dad to sign the form and then quickly disappeared out the door. The other lady stayed to chat. She spoke a lot of sense. She'd seen it all before. She spoke about what each of us was going through, what battles we all faced as individuals. When she mentioned that Dad would be thinking along the lines of 'I'm glad I've got it and not any of my other family members', it struck a chord with him and he sat upright. He seemed ready to fight.

"That's what Mari said when she was just 14." Mum said.

We fumbled our way out of the hospital, having got lost on the way out. We passed empty rooms with empty beds. In my mind's eye, I could see people curled up in those beds, and the people sat around them worried and helpless. But we soon passed a notice board full of colourful 'Thank you' cards.

"See? These are all the cards that people have sent in to say thank you for fixing them." Mum pointed out. "And they never mentioned anything about your hair falling out either." she added.

"She probably thought that that would have been a waste of a sentence with the amount of hair I've got left." quipped Dad.

Knowing that today was over, another day done, Dad had a bit of chipper about him as he headed to his car. I could sense a feeling of fight coming from his soul.

Chemo started the next morning. He was going to need that fight.

8 IRISH MARMALADE AND IRISH CRISPS

Wednesday 11th July 2012

It was a fairly early drive to pick up the gang. I'd dropped Clare off at work in the city centre for 9am and headed out in the mellow July sun. With all the serfs in work turning the heavy cogs of commerce, it was now time for the oldies to come out of hiding in their bungalows and tootle around the roads.

I stopped off in Asda on the way. I'd heard that they were doing a line of Irish foods. Mum was fascinated with anything Irish. Every other sentence would normally be about an Irish person, or a time when she was in Ireland. There wasn't that much choice on the shelves but I did pick up some Tayto crisps, some Irish marmalade and some coffee from Bewleys, the world-famous coffee shop that had now closed its doors. Mum had spent many rainy Dublin days there.

The house was silent when I arrived. I wasn't sure that anyone was in fact there. I found Dad first, who had retreated to his settee in the middle room. He was sat there in silence with no light on. I think he was worried about the chemo.

Mum was sat in the back garden, having a fag and also looking into space. Her face lit up when she saw the goodies I was holding in my arms. I put the kettle on and made us all a cup of Bewley's coffee to sharpen our heads. We needed it.

The cancer hospital was busy once again. Its waiting room was more like a train station. Unfortunately, Dad's chemo wasn't ready so we popped to a nearby Tesco where we picked up some sandwiches, crisps and chocolate. We sat in a nearby park to eat them. We always seemed to be waiting. And eating.

I lay on the grass and looked up at the sky. The weather really couldn't make its mind up. Half the sky was dazzling blue and sunshine. The other was an angry-looking cloud.

I wasn't sure which way things were going to turn out.

As it was, the angry cloud got one over on the sunshine. The park soon became grey and spots of rain flecked the concrete paths.

We headed for the car where we finished our lunch and waited for a call from the nurse to say that the room was ready.

It took another hour.

Eventually we arrived at the room where Dad would spent the next 6 days. It felt a bit dilapidated but at least he had his own privacy. He'd like that.

A female nurse, with St Tropez skin and pink palms talked Dad through the side effects of the treatment. She went through another medical questionnaire and got him to sign another form. I sat near the window and gazed out at the rain thundering down onto the small garden area outside.

It was hard leaving Dad that evening. He was already attached to the drip that would be pumping him full of toxic chemo when we left. But Mum felt happy that at least it had all started. In her mind, the chemo would be getting to work on the cancer as we headed home once again in the rain.

Thursday 12th July 2012

"He's like a pig in shit." said Mum as I arrived back at the hospital late afternoon. I'd dropped them off earlier and had to dash off to do some work in the afternoon. Now it was time for me to go and collect them.

Dad was sat in the large armchair next to his bed. The drip was still attached and he was beaming a very large smile. Dinner was on its way. Curry followed by fruit pie. We made a sharp exit as his food arrived and we left him to it. Dad loved his food.

***

"He's being waited on hand and foot there. He's away from everyone else. He's loving it."

Mum's phone buzzed. It was Dad saying that he'd already polished off both courses. We hadn't even got out of the car park.

Later on, after I'd dropped Mum and Mari home, I drove back and parked up at some shops close to my house. I grabbed a bag of chips and sat in the car in the rain and ate them. Then I headed back in to see Dad.

***

"Good to see you Number One Son." he said (I was the eldest of the siblings).

I'd taken him some macaroons but then found he had a stash of crisps, biscuits and snacks already there. He'd even pressed his buzzer and ordered a chicken sandwich from a nurse at midnight. He was getting very assertive. But it did make me sad thinking of him sat alone in a bare room during the small hours while we were all snug in our beds.

We spoke for about an hour about family issues, the hospital and the plans for the next few days and weeks. And then it was time to go.

"Keep the door open." he said. "I like to see who goes past my room."

With no meal to distract him from me leaving, it was a case of taking a big breath, giving him a hug and walking away.

It wasn't easy. It never is.

9 VICTORIA BECKHAM AND SIR TOM JONES

Friday 13th July 2012

Knock knock.

Mum's smile soon dropped. The door to Dad's room was closed. And there was no answer.

Knock knock.

I pulled down on the heavy handle and peeped in.

The first thing I saw was Dad on the bed, his T-shirt pulled up to his neck and a big beaming smile on his face. He didn't say a word. He just lay there smiling.

"Can I help?" came a small female voice from behind the door.

"Oh sorry!" I said stepping back. The nurse came to the door.

"I'm just giving him an ECG - all routine so nothing to worry about. We'll be about ten minutes if you just want to wait in the Day Room."

In the Day Room was a large chap in a wheelchair. He was on his phone and his drip stood sentry-like next to him. He was a big man, not fat - just big. Take twenty years off him and you could have almost imagined him as a steaming man mountain on a muddy rugby pitch somewhere up the valleys; smashing through players like some strapped-up wrecking ball and heading to the pub after. But here he was, wedged into a wheelchair with nowhere to go.

Mum and I took a seat next to the signed photograph of Tom Jones and picked up some magazines. They were the usual pile of high-gloss shit.

"Aw." said Mum. "I'm just reading about how Victoria Beckham went through hell for three months after she had her baby. Look - it says here that she sat in her jogging pants and cried three months. Isn't that awful?"

"Poor dab." I said. "But nothing compared to this woman." I pointed out a photograph of a woman, posing in her bikini. Her figure was perfect. "This woman hates her body. She's going through hell. She's close to suicide."

Mum peered over.

"Aw...who is she?"

"Erm...dunno. She's off The Only Way Is Essex."

"What's that?"

"Erm...dunno."

"Aw. Poor dab."

The nurse came in.

"Ah. There you are."

Mum and I leaned forward in our seats.

"We've had a little bit of a problem I'm afraid."

We waited.

"I was trying to attach an electrode to his chest but he's just a little bit..."

We waited some more.

"Yes?" said Mum. We both braced ourselves.

"Well. He's just a little bit hairy."

Air fizzled out of our mouths like a fat balloon being let down.

"It's going to take a few more minutes as we've had to shave him."

***

I had to head off for a few hours to get some work done after we'd been in to see him. I left Mum there and went to the car.

Pulling up to the exit of the car park, I stopped to look for traffic. Leaning on a walking stick, sucking on a crinkled up cigarette was a tall man about 50 years of age. His face was yellow like a large moon, and rain was dripping off his large hooked nose. He looked at me with his sunken eyes before I pulled out and headed down the road. I had been tempted to slag him off for smoking but it dawned on me that he was probably past worrying about his health.

Smoking was probably not going to make him any worse.

***

After cramming in as much work as I could, I headed back to pick up Mum. The one thing I'd noticed about the hospital over the last few days, was that I never saw any patients. Doctors and nurses, yes, but there seemed a curious lack of patients.

Which is why it was a little surprising to see the man who'd been out smoking earlier, stood in the corridor. He was still leaning on his stick and reading something on the wall. His jeans, now several sizes too big, hung off him like they were drying on a clothes horse. He looked lost.

As I passed him, I glanced at the wall to see what he was reading. It was the wall full of thank you cards. For a split second, I imagined I was him. I felt like I'd had my soul sucked out. Here he was, probably receiving palliative care, and probably feeling cheated that others had a better outcome than him. They had all gone away now, enjoying their Friday night with family and friends. And here he was, alone, dying and lost.

Would there ever be a thank you card on the wall from this man's family? Suddenly, everything we were going through all seemed very real and in my face.

Dad's door was open this time and a sense of relief came over me. I could hear Mum and Dad talking and as I popped my head around, Dad was finishing off yet another cup of tea. His face lit up.

"I've had a poo!" he exclaimed, popping the empty cup back on the saucer.

"Well done." I said.

"I weighed 85 kilos before my shit. And now I weigh 80."

"That was hell of a shit Dad."

"I know. Tell me about it. The laxatives did their job."

"Is it on the chart?" I said, looking to the splattering of charts that were stuck to the wall.

"Not yet." said Dad, opening a KitKat and snapping it in half near his face. "It's not official yet."

For now at least, it all seemed to be going well. Dad was in good spirits, if perhaps a bit stir-crazy. He'd been sat in his chair doing the actions to Agadoo before I had arrived, and we all laughed at the newspaper reports about some female MP who'd gone off on one at the House of Commons the previous day.

It was on way home that Mum started opening up about how she was handling things. She couldn't look more than one day ahead. Another day down and we'd gotten through it - that was her way of looking at it. It was a good way.

Look too far ahead and it could all get too much.

That night in bed, I thought about Dad. I thought about the man who had been stood there looking at the thank you cards. Then I thought about having to earn some money, after watching a TV programme where a group of London plumbers revealed that they were on £150,000 a year. I worked hard and I'm sure they did too. But how can we both work just as hard and they earn so much more? Then I remembered what I'd overheard an old woman say as I passed her in the rain a few days earlier.

"Your health is your wealth." she'd said to her husband as he walked on ahead of her. I had no idea why she said it. There appeared to be no conversation going on.

But she was right. Money will get you so far but I'd rather health than wealth.

I just hoped that Dad could repay the debt he'd burdened himself with through smoking.

10 CHRISTMAS SHERRY AND THE THEATRE ROYAL

Monday 16th July 2012
Me>Dad: I'm here. Meet me out the front
Dad>Me: Awwwwwsome! On the effing dot too! See you in 5 bro!

Judging by Dad's text, he was happy to be leaving hospital. A few minutes later, he opened the back door of my car, slugged his bag in and climbed in.

"Yes!" he exclaimed and punched the air. "I'm out!"

The rain had returned once again.

"Horrible weather." I moaned as we pulled out of the car park.

"Yes. But it's sunny up here." replied Dad, pointing a finger to the temple of his head.

******December 24th 1984******

Mum's parents lived in a house up the hill opposite our house. We could see their house from ours. Mum would often ask me to look out the window to see if they were in. This particular Christmas Eve, they'd just dropped us home after Midnight Mass and Mum wanted me to make sure that they got home ok. I stood in our front room and I watched the tail lights of their Triumph Toledo as it disappeared up around the back of the hill in the dark.

At the back of our house, my parents and a few aunties and uncles were gathering around a late-night bottle of sherry. I could hear the glug-glug-glugging of the sherry being poured and the clinking of the glasses as they toasted another Christmas together. But the front room was peaceful. The coloured lights on the tree were as silent as stars. I leant down to the stereo player that was on the bottom shelf and pressed 'Play' on the tape deck. I think it was the Coventry Carol that came on. I moved over to the bay window and looked out.

It was a cold hard night. The concrete lampposts stood guarding the steel streets but across the way came the warm glow of light from my grandparents' living room window. I could see them, taking off their coats, and then embracing and exchanging a kiss under the mistletoe that was hanging from the light fixture. Even from the distance that I was away from them, and despite the silence of the night outside the window, I could sense their love for each other. And it was at that moment, while I felt like the town was settling down for the night, that I felt that for once, all was well with the world.

I eventually went to bed. I woke up several times but by 6am, Santa had been. All I had to do was wriggle my toes. The soft crackling of the wrapping paper was all I needed to hear. In the cold light of morning, it felt like we were pretending it was Christmas, acting it out almost. We'd go to church but I was always secretly glad when that was over. It was only when we got back home, with Dad there in his apron, and a waft of warm food to greet us at the door, did it really feel like Christmas Day.

We'd usually have a party in the evening and Boxing Day, we'd all head to the 'club' after. New Year's Eve came round soon enough but it never had the magic that Christmas had. Mum would talk about the wild New Year's Eve parties that took place 'down *the club': "You wouldn't want to be down there - everyone snogs everyone else's face off." she once told me. As a young teenager, I couldn't wait for the day to turn 18 so I could get myself in. Instead, I had to stay home and sip Bailey's with Dad. It was no bad thing. We'd wrap up warm and head up the hill. We'd sit on the bench that overlooked Barry and the docks and watch the last of the fireworks fade into last year. The ships would still be droning their horns in celebration as we made our way home.*

******

"It feels weird being back home." he said as we made our way nearer to Dad's house. "They've even resurfaced this road...I'll have to drive along this later just for a novelty."

We spoke about the treatment he'd been having at the hospital.

"I haven't felt sick. My hair hasn't fallen out. I haven't had any mouth ulcers." he said.

"I've been blessed."

In a way, he was right. There was still a long way to go. When I thought back to my sister Mari being ill, it was hard sometimes to open the door and see her lying there like some archaeological find on her bed. Dad had seemed to get away with it so far and considering he only had to have two chemo treatments, he was feeling pretty pleased with himself.

Mum had sent us a text to say that she'd put the kettle on as we pulled up outside the house. Perfect timing to go with the stack of pepper pasties we'd bought. The house had been made cosy. The coal fire was hissing into life and Dad took his shoes off and picked up the papers that were waiting for him at the side of the settee.

As I headed back home, I had to make a detour which took me past our local cinema. Like many in the town, I'd go there as a kid. Although it had been threatened with demolition for many years, it came as a shock to see the long yellow arm of a crane slashing its way through its walls as I passed. Peering in to its pink innards, I could make out a dark empty chasm, now exposed to the rain, where once fathers, grandfathers and great grandfathers would try their charm on their ladies. A room full of memories escaping into the cold grey day.

"I thought you'd be there forever." I said to myself.

'It's only when those things are threatened with their very existence that we sit up and take notice.' I thought.

11 BARRY BUTTRILLS AND THE OLYMPICS

Tuesday 31st July 2012

Mari> Sam Hey you, I was thinking today of when I had my operation in Birmingham & all I can remember is you holding my hand for ages. I just wanted to say thank you for making me laugh when all I wanted to do was cry, I miss you xxxxxx

It was four years ago to the day that my kid sister was having a life-saving operation to have her cancer-riddled knee taken out.

She was 14 when she was told that she had it. Except she wasn't really told as such. It sort of slipped out from a bone surgeon as we sat in a shitty cubicle in A&E. My GP cousin, who had turned up, luckily knew what an osteosarcoma was and tried to let us all know gently that it was cancer, by asking the doctor:

"So what's treatment likely to be? Chemo?"

We all looked at each other. Mari let out one of her nervous laughs. Mum and Dad bolted out for a cigarette. My friend Danielle was stood the other side of the bed to me. It was up to us to explain to Mari what was happening and what the treatment would likely to entail.

That was hard. Telling your kid sister that she was going to lose her beautiful hair as well as having to endure all the shit that came with it.

It was also a hard seven months watching my sister being ground into the hospital bedding with all the chemo. It was hard watching her immediately after her operation to replace her knee. To be able to leave the Birmingham Children's Hospital, she had to prove to the doctors that she could walk up the long disabled access ramp that led to the canteen. It took her a while and her poor pale legs were quivering. But she wanted to go home. She wanted her own room, Mum's food and her own telly. She did in the end.

It was in the early hours of January 1st, 2009 that she finished her chemo. She went on to finish her GCSEs, complete her A-levels, enrolled in a posh London University and got herself a 6'3 Marine boyfriend. If someone had told us that in the summer of 2008, I'd have kissed them.

******June 1986******

Summers always seemed longer and hotter when I was a kid. I could always smell summer coming when I'd be sat daydreaming in school lessons. At break times, we'd head out to the field and sit and eat our warm sandwiches. School always smelt of cut grass in the summer.

At the weekends, Dad would take us three brothers 'up the Butts', a large recreational field at the top of our town. We'd pack a football, a rugby ball and some squash into a plastic bag on Saturday afternoons while Mum's sisters came round to talk at each other. We'd head out, up the hill, stopping off at the corner shop at the top. There, Dad would buy us bubble gum, World Cup ones because they came with stickers of players, and Dad would treat himself to a pack of Trebor mints. Then we'd head silently on, past the sleeping souls in the cemetery and on to the playing fields.

The Butts was always empty. Whoever was carrying the football as we stepped onto the grass would boot the ball as far as they could. If it was still football season, we'd take our pick of dozens of posts. If it was the height of summer, we'd use makeshift goalposts from our plastic bag and our jumpers.

Sometimes we played the entire full-length pitch. Two-on-two. It was usually Dad and Dylan, my youngest brother, against me and Dan. Dylan was very small and I'd stay in goal. Dan would take a few minutes to reach Dad, who'd then launch the ball way over Dan's head and down on to me. When we got bored of that, we'd play 'Whoever scores goes in goal' which was a bit naff as being in goal was crap. I'd end up pulling the gaffer tape off the posts while I waited for my brothers' little legs to carry him down the length of the pitch.

Those summer afternoons seemed endless. We had no worries. Not a care in the world. The only thing we'd be concerned about was whether the squash would hold out. If we were lucky, we'd head up to the Spar, at the other end of the field. Dad would buy us cold cans of Quatro. I always wanted the cardboard periscope that was on one of the racks. I never got one though.

The fields seemed to seethe and whisper as it cooled in late simmering of the afternoon. We'd pack up our stuff and head home, tired but happy. At home, we would have a bath, our tea and a night watching The A-Team, Streethawk, Family Fortunes and 3-2-1, smelling of Matey.

******

Wednesday 1st August 2012

In the few weeks in between treatments, the sun had finally broken through.

"We're quite full at the moment so I'll just lead you to your room." said the nurse. She led us down the corridor and into a room with three other beds. Dad's face dropped as he slung his bag onto the bed. In the corner of the room, lying on the bed, was a man with a beard and a small wife.

We waited to be attended to. A skinny man came in and sat on one of the other beds. He was curled right over on the end of his bed, trying to open a packet of mints. He looked like a question mark. I could see in Dad's face that this was not what he was expecting. What had happened to the private en-suite rooms?

Mum tried to lighten the mood by handing me the birthday cards and gifts she'd brought in a plastic bag. A bottle of wine and some cards. We spoke about how fast time goes. Mum told me about how Nan used to still say "I'm still waiting to have a jelly all to myself." I had no birthday jelly today.

After an hour or so, I headed over to Danielle's house. She wanted to take me for a coffee for my birthday. But she had been under an enormous amount of pressure with events in her life too. Nothing seemed to be going right for her. She cried into her coffee. It was sad to see such a usually strong person being reduced to tears. I gave her a hug but left her with a heavy heart. I knew she'd have to go back to her life and carry on her hard slog.

It wasn't the birthday I'd been wanting. My only birthday wish, if I believed in them, would be to make all the problems that my friends and family had, go away.

Thursday 2nd August 2012

I arrived in hospital the next day to find Dad's bed empty. It was all made up and Dad's belongings weren't there.

After some searching, I found him, sat like a king, in his own personal room. He was eating as usual, and watching some rowers at the Olympics on his tiny telly.

"There you are."

"Ah hello."

"How come you're in here?" I asked.

"I asked to be moved."

"You ok?"

"Yeah. Well...sort of." said Dad. He waited till I'd taken my seat.

"I had a bit of a low moment yesterday." he confessed.

"How come?"

"The doctors told me that the tumour hasn't shrunk."

"How do they know?"

"From the scans."

He asked me what I made of it all. In our heads, we justified why it appeared not to have shrunk. It was still a worry though, no matter what we said to make it seem better.

I wandered down the corridor to get some air. The door to the room next to Dad's was wide open. The guy was fast asleep with the portable TV screen right up to his nose. He wasn't even roused by the excitable commentator as British rowers headed for another Olympic gold.

In the room next to them was an older couple. They were clutching onto each other. They looked scared and lonely; probably the first time they'd been there. It reminded me that we weren't the only family going through it.

Monday 6th August 2012

Dad had finished his second bout of chemo and was heading home. What I found strange was that the sun always came out when Dad was on his way home. He wound down the window as I drove along. He had his head hanging half out like some kind of excited dog. He was finding it strange adapting to the sunlight.

He had two weeks ahead of him now of doing nothing. Nothing but worry anyway. It'd be a few weeks before he started the gruelling six-week course of radiotherapy. We thought we'd had it hard so far. Truth be told, we'd had it easy up until now.

12 HOT SAND AND COWBOY HATS

Tuesday 18th August 2012

The last time I'd laid on a beach was probably over ten years ago. The beach at Barry Island was pretty deserted, which was odd considering that the sun was out for a change. Mum, Mari and I headed to the middle of the beach, put down three towels and unfurled ourselves on the hot sand.

I pulled down my cap over my face and for the first time in years, I lay there and just listened to the soft breath of the sea, and felt the breeze skipping over me. The sun was sizzling my skin like a bubbling sausage. I'd forgotten what that felt like. In my private world of the inside of my cap, I remembered the days we'd spend there as kids, when the days were long, hot and carefree.

Afterwards, we headed up for an ice-cream. While we waited for our lift, I peered over the railings and into the wasteland that once used to be Barry Island Butlins. Years ago, thousands would pass through those gates. Today, there was a grizzly mother and her two kids sniffing around the gate.

"Thomas!" snarled the woman. "Where you going?"

The boy, probably about six years old was hot and sweaty. His face was one big beef-red huff.

"I want to look in the shop."

"Well don't be long."

He disappeared into the shop, only to reappear a few minutes later with a cowboy hat on his head. He hadn't even taken the cardboard rim off it and was wearing the hat, label and all.

"What you bloody got there?" shrieked the mother. If Steptoe had a sister, this was her.

"A nat."

"Well you can bloody take that right back now and get your bloody money back. I'm not having you wasting money on that shit." She spoke so fast that her words tripped over each other.

The boy's face dropped as the mother headed over to him and dragged him back into the shop. Dad arrived and as we pulled away, Thomas, mother and sister were coming back out of the shop. The hat was still on his head.

13 LUCY'S LEGACY

Tuesday 21st August 2012

I'd put the bins out and locked up. I'd fetched a glass of water and sat at my computer to log off. Bed beckoned.

The last thing to do was switch my computer off. My Facebook page was up and it was always worth a casual browse to see what was going on in the world. There was the usual bollocks - someone who'd had too much to drink. There was the whinger. Then there was the one who seemed grossly in love with someone they'd only just met.

Scrolling down, I'd seen my friend Kevin had posted a picture of him and my friend Lucy. It never ceased to amaze me how many times two friends of mine were also friends with each other without me knowing. Kevin was dressed as a vampire and Lucy - just vampish. Gorgeous girl. I was just about to click off when I saw what Kevin had written:

RIP Lucy.

My finger hovered over my mouse. I didn't understand. I didn't want to click on Lucy's profile. But I had to.

******March 2002******

Back then, my life was a bit of a mess. I had money worries. I had no identity. Worse still, I had no direction.

I ended up working in a shitty call centre. We'd be the people who'd tell you where the nearest hairdresser or cement mixer was. Yep. We were the really important people.

We'd work long shifts. Every time we got up from our desks, we'd have to log it and be signed off. Taking a piss wasn't as easy as you thought.

We had breaks. By law. Back then, we had a smoking room – a small room in the middle of the building, high up in the Cardiff skyline. It stank of course, but it was our only escape from the misery of the call centre.

It was late one night, in that stinking room, that I met a girl called Lucy. She too was from Barry, I found out. She was one of twins. She was always smiling, despite the desperate situation we found ourselves in. She was small, but determined to change the world.

I'd seen it all before of course. Call centres were often the watering hole for lost souls wanting to do something big. Except Lucy did do something big. We left the call centre and went our separate ways. I drifted for a few more years. But Lucy did what she said she was going to do - she changed the world.

It was only a few years later when I found her on Facebook that I realised what she had achieved since we'd last seen each other. She'd headed up a charity that was making a real difference to people in Africa. Whereas I was donating a fiver here and there on my mobile phone to Comic Relief, this girl was on the ground, meeting the people whose lives she was changing for the better.

I was jealous. Not in a nasty way. I was jealous of her bravery. I was jealous of her passion. I was jealous of her vision. Whereas I talked it, she did it.

To the people she met, she changed their world. For the better.

Facebook brings both pleasure and pain. Last night, I found out that my beautiful friend is no longer with us. I can still hear her voice. I can still hear her laugh. To those closer to her, it must feel like the end of their world. Life has given us someone who has inspired. She'll be missed. Her Facebook page won't be updated again. Her last status said that she was off to see some hippos. Strangely enough, I had been watching a programme about African elephants before I headed to bed last night. They focused on one matriarch in particular, a beautiful and intelligent creature, who put her family and extended family first and inspired a generation. And that's what Lucy did. To all the people she met, she touched their hearts and made them think again.

******

Tuesday 28th August 2012

Dad and I were heading into hospital. It'd been a few weeks since we were last there but Dad had to go in for a 24 hour stay and a blast of chemo. He'd been there earlier in the day for his first dose of radiotherapy. He'd been sat there with the mesh mask they'd made for him to get his first hit. Then nothing.

"Sorry. The machine's not working."

They tried again a few hours later with a bit more success.

Dad seemed a little apprehensive in the car. I think he was worried about my mum. There were a lot of things going on within the family that weren't helping. If ever there was a bad time for several family crises to happen at once, this was it.

"You can just drop me off. I know the score now."

I watched him disappear in to the hospital, small bag in hand.

I sighed before pulling away and leaving him there. We now had six weeks of radiotherapy to get through. Then we'd know if the pain of the last few months had worked.

14 MINCED BEEF PIES AND FINAL DEMANDS

Wednesday 29th August 2012

It was the usual pick-up at the hospital. Dad reappeared still clutching his bag. The only thing missing from it was a multi-pack of KitKats that my mum had sneaked in there.

"How are you, number one son?"

"I'm ok. Tired and stressed with work and the house move and all that. But I'm ok ta. How did it go?"

"Fine. All went to plan. You had anything to eat?"

"No."

"Mm. Nor me. I had to turn down a pork dinner for this and I'm starving."

"Pepper pasties? They'll be doing your favourite mince beef and gravy pies today."

Dad almost lost himself for a minute.

"Oh God yes! I hope to God that they've got pies in today. I want to eat and eat and EAT!" He pretended to shovel food into his mouth like some sort of demented Cookie Monster. I think he was glad to be out.

The conversation down the M4 soon turned to the next six weeks. I'd told him that I'd planned them all on a chart, right down to meals so that I could fit all the running around in with my work. I'd feel out of control otherwise.

"I had to grow up when first my father died, and then my mother." said Dad. He'd never spoken before about losing his dad. Mum had told me that she'd been working in a shoe shop back in the mid seventies, when Dad came in like a whirlwind, long coat flapping behind him, to tell my mum what had happened. This vision had stuck with me for a long time. How hard must that have been? A newly-married young man with kids, losing his dad like that. I didn't want to think about it.

"I had to grow up pretty quickly." said Dad. "I had kids to feed."

We spoke about taking life's responsibilities seriously. We swapped stories of hiding water bills, stuffing final demands down the back of cupboards and putting off telling people bad news until the last possible minute. Neither of us were perfect, but we'd both learnt our lessons along the way.

We pulled up at Waitrose petrol station to load up on coal. Dark storm clouds were rumbling in from the west as we filled the car boot with bags of coal. We picked up some pasties from the bakery and managed to get in the house just before the heavens opened. For ten or fifteen minutes, I lost myself in my pasties, a cup of tea and a copy of the South Wales Echo before picking up my keys and leaving for home.

I stopped to wave goodbye from the garden path. As I did, the grey smoky haze of the coal burning fire drifted down off the rain-sheened roof and wrapped its arms tight around me.

Autumn was coming.

15 SECRET BEERS AND THE UPHILL STRUGGLE

******Christmas Day 1993******

It wasn't very often that our large family would be in one place at one time so we always looked forward to Christmas Day evenings at our house. As kids, it was the only time of year we got to see our aunties and uncles drunk which we found amusing. It also meant that us kids seemed to have more authority. We were the ones that took charge of proceedings. Mari, our little baby sister was tucked up safely far away in the back bedroom of the house. We'd occasionally hear her stir on the baby monitor that we had on the mantelpiece, and the room full of people would fall silent for a moment.

"Shhhh. Baby monitor!!!" said Mum sternly. We all fell silent and watched the monitor. No idea what we were expecting to see.

"Ok. All clear." said Mum after hearing Mari settle herself down. The party resumed.

We'd had two board games the previous Christmas. One was called Brit Quiz and the other was called Dare. Brit Quiz always came first before Dare was cracked open after a few beers.

One of my brother's friends James was hammered before 6pm. He was around 19 years of age and always seemed to be drunk. We'd often see him at the Friars night-club down at Barry Island, off his face and curled up asleep in a ball in the middle of the dance floor.

"I've got a Bong Crisby Christmas CD in the

glove compartment of my car! I'll just go and get it!" he mumbled before falling out of the patio doors, never to be seen again. It was one less drunk for Dad to worry about. He hated people in his house.

My brother Dylan picked up a Dare card and read it out.

"Right! Brian! You need to do 50 press-ups." Dylan had lied of course. The card's instructions were to do ten press-ups but Dylan knew that Brian, who at around 5'3 and rather round, would struggle.

"On your knuckles!" added Dylan. The kids were in charge tonight.

"Right! I'm there! I'm Brian the Lion - strong as iron!" shouted Brian before rolling up his sleeves and getting down on his hands and knees. We all counted out the press-ups while he got going. By seven, his face was turning red and a ring of sweat was rising up his paper Christmas hat.

"8.9.10." Brian started trembling and growling.

"Come on Brian! We need these points!"

"11.12.13..."

Brian's eyes were popping. His brown Clarks loafers creaked every time he lowered his heavy frame to the carpet.

"He's going to have a heart attack!" someone cried.

"Come on Brian you big girl!" came another voice. "Come on!!!!!"

Despite all his shaking and sweating, Brian incredibly managed to get to 40 and was still going. His red-raw knuckles were buckling and cracking.

"Come on Brian!! Only ten more left!"

Dylan, realising that Brian had defied his instructions, stood up.

"I forgot to say," he said, holding up the card "...with someone on your back!"

And with that, Dylan jumped on Brian's back.

"Yay!" cried Dylan, sat astride the fallen beast. "Another failure! I'm off to get a drink!"

Dylan was enjoying his evening. He headed to the empty kitchen to see what he could drink and get away with while all the grown-ups were drunk. The kitchen table was strewn with empty beer cans, some used as ash-trays, half-empty wine bottles and plastic six-pack rings. The fridge offered up nothing of interest so Dylan quietly climbed the stairs and tip-toed down the long passage towards the back bedroom where Mari lay sleeping. He knew that Dad had a secret stash of beer hiding under Mari's cot.

The door creaked open.

"Sssssh!" said Dad. He was already there, sat on the floor, enjoying a sneaky warm Spar Pilsner lager.

"Got any beer?"

Dad exploded as quietly as he could.

"For God's sake. You as well? I'm sick of these bastards coming to my house, eating my food, drinking my beer."

Downstairs, Mum shushed the crowd in the living room.

"Shhhh. Baby monitor!!!" The noise subsided to a hush. We could hear Dad and Dylan talking. We all sat there, listening to the conversation that was taking place far away in the back bedroom of the house.

"I only want the one can." said Dylan.

"Greedy bastards the lot of them. All I wanted was a quiet Christmas. All my food's gone, my drink's gone. That's why I've had to put a secret slab here under the bed. Why can't they all just fuck off and leave me to my own house?"

Us kids watched as our aunties and uncles sat heads down, peering into their flat beer. Brian took *off his damp Christmas hat and stuffed it into the pocket of his tweed jacket. Within a couple of minutes, they'd all put their coats on and headed out into the cold Christmas night.*

Dad was up early the next morning, slugging out the bins full of empty cans and bottles. He hadn't meant to cause offence and protested his innocence to Mum as he struggled down the garden path with the heavy bags.

"I was only joking." he said. "I knew they'd all be able to hear me!" But Mum didn't buy it.

As he passed James's car, he placed his bags on the floor and peered in.

James was sat in the passenger seat, head bowed asleep, and with his hand still in his glove compartment, clutching a Bing Crosby Christmas CD.

******

Tuesday 4th September 2012

ME: Hi Mum. It's me.
MUM: Oh hiya love....you ok?
ME: Yeah. Fine ta. You ok? You sound knackered.
MUM: I'm...I'm...hang on....[catching her breath] I'm on my way home with the shopping.
ME: Up that bloody hill?
MUM: Yeah....phew. Hang on. Let me put the shopping down. Ok. Free now.
ME: I was just phoning to see whether you need a lift to the hospital today.
MUM: He should be ok. He wants to keep on going as long as he can.
ME: Ok. How's he feeling in himself?

MUM: Well the sickness is starting to kick in now. He's started his anti-sickness drugs. He's completely gone off his food.

ME: So no more pepper pasties then?

MUM: No. And I know how much of a comfort food it is to him.

ME: Well I guess we've had a pretty easy ride of it all up until now.

MUM: Yeah...I'm going to carry on walking as it's starting to rain.

ME: Shall I call you when you get home?

MUM: No. It's ok. Nearly there.

ME: Well I'll stay on stand-by if you need me. Are you coping ok?

MUM: Not really. I'm feeling like Stretch Armstrong. I don't think anyone understands the stress I'm under. People are asking favours of me left, right and centre and I'm finding it hard to cope. I was physically sick with stress and worry yesterday.

ME: [sighs] Well you know I'm here if you need me for anything.

MUM: I know. And we appreciate it [sound of rustling of bags] Home now. [sighs]

ME: Good. Put the kettle on and get yourself some rest.

MUM: I will. I'm just looking out the window. While you're there, I wanted to ask if you knew anyone who does guttering? Mine's broken and I'm worried that the water will start coming in the house.

ME: I'll ask arou...

MUM: I've got to go. There's a cat in my garden. He's looking me right in the eye and shitting on my lawn. Bye.

[click]

16 HOMETOWN GLORY AND THE OAK TREE

Wednesday 5th September 2012

I'd been on the phone to my sister Beti for two hours. Normally the one who held everything together, I think that things were beginning to get to her now too. We spoke about how Dad was now starting to feel the pace, how Mum was struggling to keep up and how as a family, we all needed to pull together. But my brother Dylan was close to breaking point and had gone missing. We were all worried. It wasn't fair on our parents. Mum was watching her soul mate stumble. She needed our help. Dad wasn't going to be able to help her this time.

When Beti and I finished talking, I lay on my bed.

Thoughts swirled around my head, lapping and diving over each other, each of them clamouring for my attention. For the first time, I felt scared and alone.

I nodded off slightly and woke to find myself late to pick up my wife from town.

"Shit."

I quickly threw some clothes on and jumped in the car.

For the first time in months, I felt like I needed some music in the car. I found a CD down the side of the door and slid it in, not knowing what it was. It didn't really matter. As it was, Adele's Hometown Glory came on as I raced into town. I'm not one of her biggest fans but the music seemed appropriate somehow.

   As I sped into town, I wondered where my brother was. I wondered if he was safe. The sad piano chords moved me and I felt strangely distant from my home town as the evening sun dappled the road laid out ahead of me. The people flashed by - the tourists with the bumbags, the couples heading out for a meal, the mother with her child on a bike, the worker heading home from work, the jogger, the drunk, the girl with the floaty dress. I'm sure they had their problems too but for me right now, my mountain seemed far too big, too huge. But we had to come together and fight. We had to.

Shows that we ain't gonna take it
Shows that we ain't gonna stand shit
Shows that we are united

'Pressure makes diamonds.' I thought.

Thursday 6th September 2012

Beti>Me I've booked Dylan a bus ticket up to my house. Can you make sure he gets on it please? xx
Me>Beti Aye xx

I hadn't seen Dad for a few weeks now and the talk of him losing weight made me nervous. I didn't want to see him ill. Mum was waiting at the back door when I arrived at their house. Stepping inside, there sat in a chair in the corner of the dining room was my brother Dylan. He looked drawn and gaunt. I gave him a big hug and could smell last night's alcohol on his clothes. In a way, it was a relief that he'd been drinking. It explained his ramblings on the phone the previous night. I'd gone to bed convinced that his head had gone 'pop'.

"Want some gammon and egg?" asked Mum from the kitchen.

"Yes please." replied Dylan. I thought he could do with some food.

After he'd eaten, I took him to his house to pick up some clothes. There, he headed straight to the garden, sat cross-legged on a wooden chair, and lit up a cigarette. His hands were shaking.

"What are you going to do?" I asked him.

"Dunno."

He sucked his cigarette hard, staring at the fading flowers in the garden before dropping the cigarette to the floor and stubbing it out with his desert boot.

"Let's go."

I had planned on giving him a pep talk in the car on the way to the bus stop in town but I think we were both too tired. He reached into his rucksack and pulled out a Bob Dylan CD.

"I appreciate this. I couldn't stay with mother and father. Seeing Dad ill takes me over the edge. I can't cope with it."

He popped the CD into the car stereo with his shaky hands.

"Have you heard this one? Mississippi by Bob Dylan. There's a line in there which says 'Only one thing I did wrong - stayed in Mississippi a day too long.' I guess that's what I did." he said.

Half hour later, we were stood on the bus stop outside Cardiff's City Hall. Dylan's eyes were lingering on the other passengers waiting for the bus. He looked worried.

"I hope she doesn't sit next to me." he said.

I looked over to see a woman, late fifties,

wearing a scraggly grey T-shirt and grey leggings. Her gut was something of a landslide and a crooked cigarette dangled precariously from her dry chapped lips.

"I'm sure she'll be alright." I said. "She's travelling alone so you won't have to listen to her."

"I'm more worried about the smell." he replied.

Having waved my brother off, it was time to head down to the Vale to say goodbye to another friend. Hundreds gathered underneath a large oak tree in the middle of a sunny meadow to say their farewells to our friend Lucy. Her funeral was being held here in Wales, but in small villages across the world, others gathered to remember her too. That's how far her inspiration and magic stretched.

One by one, members of Lucy's family stood at the microphone to say a few words. First her parents. I couldn't imagine the pain they were going through. Then her brother-in-law. A poem about the bird-watching adventures they used to get up to together. High above us, in the shimmering late summer sky, a lone swallow looped and dived. I think I was the only one who noticed.

Then Lucy's boyfriend spoke. A beautiful man with a beautiful voice. He held his scribbled speech in his trembling hand and the sellotape that delicately held it together as it fluttered in the summer breeze, did little to hold back his emotions. He was a broken man.

Hannah, Lucy's twin sister, spoke wonderfully about her 'twin egg'. She read out a poem about life's priorities, and how everyone should make the most of their lives:

"Plant seeds and bulbs in your garden. Do not wait for someone to bring you flowers." she said. Members of the family, each and every one of them brave, brave, brave beyond words.

Then they lowered Lucy into the meadow forever. It broke my heart.

After we'd all said our goodbyes, we headed back to our cars, leaving Lucy there in that sunny field, under the oak tree and a lone swallow that looped and dived.

There was a bit of a get-together at Porthceri Country Park in the long evening sun afterwards. A part of the field had been sectioned off with bunting and fairy lights. There were food tents. There was music playing, people laughing, drinking and eating. Most of all, there was magic and love.

On my way home, I passed Mum, Dad and Mari as they were heading home from the hospital and Dad's radiotherapy treatment. They all waved frantically, all smiles. Although the afternoon had been a beautifully painful one, it had taken me away from the day-to-day worries.

It was as I pulled up at my house, and the engine was quietly chugging over, that I realised my phone was ringing. I looked at my phone. It was Clare, my wife.

"You ok love?" I said.

"Hiya love." she replied. "No. We've got a problem."

17 PUSS AND THE BOOTS

Tuesday 11th September 2012

Moving house was the last thing I wanted to do with everything else going on, but we'd seen a lovely little place a few streets away and decided to go for it. It wasn't often that nice places popped up for rent.

I pulled the car up at the new place. Halfway in and halfway out of our front door was our new settee at a very peculiar angle. One of the deliverymen was on his knees, trousers halfway down the crack of his arse, trying to peer under the sofa.

I got out the car.

"You ok?"

The deliveryman shook his head.

"Yewer never going to get that in there butt. Too big see? Can you take the window out?"

"Erm. No. It's a rented property and this is our first day here. The landlord's not going to be happy if I start taking her windows out."

"Ah, it's easy mun." He raised his dry, cracked hands to the window. "Puff, puff puff." he said, pointing to several places along the window frame and pretending to shoot them with a gun. "A big screwdriver, wang it in, pop it out, Bob's yer uncle."

"Hm. No. They'll have to go back." I said. I looked at Clare. She bit her bottom lip. It was a problem. But it was nothing compared to some of the things we'd been through these last few months. It could be sorted.

As evening fell, I sat on the doorstep of our old place and ate the half-eaten trifle that was the last surviving thing in the fridge. It had been a long hard day cleaning and moving house but we were more or less done. From underneath a nearby bush emerged our little feline friend. He'd often pop out when we pulled up in the car and liked to welcome us home. We had no idea who he belonged to but he often made himself at home in our house. But this time, he seemed to sense that we were leaving for good. He brushed past me on the doorstep and headed inside to see my wife. Purring and pawing, he didn't leave Clare's side. Then he tried sitting on the settee. He went upstairs. He tried every trick he could think of to stop us leaving. Clare couldn't stop her tears.

But it was time to go, time to move on. We scooped him up and locked the house behind us for the last time. Our cat friend looked at us for a while, then turned and headed away.

'Things never stay the same.' I thought. My eyes lingered on him as he disappeared into the dusk-dark distance of the street. To find a new adventure. With new friends.

I recalled a slogan written on the hospital wall when we took Dad into hospital for the first time back in May.

"Change is the law of life. And those who look only to the past or present are certain to miss the future." I think it was JFK who said it.

I thought of Dad. And I thought of my family's future. Would it be the same? Or would it change?

For my lifetime, Dad had been invincible. I was hoping that his invincibility would see him through this.

It had been a long hot summer. We hadn't seen a drop of rain for about two months.

My day job was answering telephone calls in an office down at Barry Docks. The office was situated in an old railway building that had no proper ventilation. I was glad to get out at 6pm, just to get some fresh air.

"Do you want a lift?" said Clive, my workmate as he stepped into his BMW.

"Nah, I'm fine." I replied.

"Looks like rain finally." he said, pointing to the darkening skies in the east.

"Nah, I'm fine honest thanks."

Clive got in his car, started his engine and pulled away. He stopped as he passed me and wound down his window.

"Don't get struck by lightning mind." he said. "Big storm rolling in. They've forecast thunder. There was a bloke who was jogging down Porthcawl promenade a few years ago. He got struck by lightning and literally disappeared. All that was left was a pair of steaming trainers!"

I laughed. So did Clive.

"Sounds like something out of a cartoon!" I replied.

"Yeah, well it wasn't funny for the guy down at Porthcawl!" chuckled Clive before driving off in a cloud of dust.

I arrived home just as the black clouds were about to burst over our house. Clive wasn't wrong. Within minutes, the foundations of the house began to shake.

"Bloody hell!" shouted Mum, who had her

head down and came running in from the back garden. The hot summer evening had soon turned into armageddon. Everything went black. The house rumbled.

"I hope your father's going to be ok." said Mum.

"Why?"

"He's walking home in this."

I, for one was worried, especially after what Clive had told me about the jogger down at Porthcawl. Dad often walked home from work and he usually got home just before me. I leapt upstairs to look out of the front bedroom window. I couldn't see far down the street but I could at least see if his arrival was imminent.

It wasn't. He was nowhere to be seen.

As I stepped out of the front bedroom, I happened to glance out of the window on the landing that was situated right over the front door. In that instant, the whole window lit up like some giant flash bulb. Before I had time to duck, the entire house shook. The wall of sound was instant and earth-shaking. It was like a bomb had gone off. The shock of it threw me against the wall at the back of the landing. The 'blast' didn't last long but my ears were ringing. I felt like we'd been depth-charged.

"Everyone ok?" shouted Mum from downstairs.

"Yes." I shouted back. "I just hope that no-one was stood by the front door. Otherwise they would have had it good and proper."

It was a few seconds before I realised what I'd said. If I hadn't seen Dad walking to the house, perhaps he'd been stood at the front door waiting to be let in.

My feet didn't touch the stairs. I flew. Within a matter of seconds, I was stood on the inside of the front door. I could feel the rain slamming into it. It took me a few seconds to rip off the locks and bolts that had been strapped across the door. Then I took a big breath and opened it.

I'd often heard of the expression 'heart in your mouth', but until this point in time, I'd never known what it meant. I did now. Every last drop of blood in my body dropped to my feet. I couldn't believe my eyes. There, stood on the doorstep, facing inwards, was an empty pair of Dad's boots.

I couldn't speak. I couldn't do anything. I wanted to shout out to Mum but I didn't know how to. All that was left of Dad were two unlaced, sodden boots.

I must have been stood there for a few minutes. My feet were getting wet. I didn't care. But then I heard squelching footsteps approaching. I looked up to see Dad, running up the garden path, clutching his jacket and holding a newspaper over his head.

"Quick! Let me in!" he shouted.

I stood to one side, still in shock. Dad dashed in, bringing in the wet and the cold. He shook the water from his head. I was happy to see him, but even so, I was angry.

"What the frig are those boots doing there?" I shouted.

"Where?" Dad looked around to see the pair of boots still pointing inwards.

"Oh them. They got dog shit all over them." he said, disappearing down the corridor to the kitchen to see what Mum had made for tea.

******

Saturday 22nd September 2012

MUM: Hiya. You ok?
ME: Yeah, good ta.
MUM: You still got that cold?
ME: Sort of. Hard to shift. Been a pain in the arse to be honest as I haven't been able to see Dad for a few weeks now.
MUM: Well do you think you'll be able to help out again? Mari is back in university now which means she won't be able to give us lifts into hospital every day.
ME: Yeah should be fine. Monday the first day - you need a lift?
MUM: Yep. We've only got two weeks left of his treatment now so hopefully, we shouldn't need you after that.
ME: Ok, no problem. Pick you up at one?
MUM: Lovely. Thanks love.
ME: Ok. See you soon. Love you.
MUM: Love you too.

In many ways, I'd been given a break away from Dad's illness but now it was my turn to step back into the fray. With just over two weeks left of treatment, these were the days we weren't looking forward to when we were sat in that small hot room back in June. It wasn't the illness that was making him ill. It was the bloody treatment. His planned chemo had been delayed too because his bloods were low. I was just hoping we could see these last two weeks out without any hiccups.

18 FOR ONE NIGHT ONLY

Tuesday 25th September 2012

"Now Thursdays have always been orange and Saturdays have always been red. Like a big red balloon."

Mum was going off on one of her little jaunts down memory lane while we headed back into hospital. Dad was sat in the back quietly, duffle coat on and a scarf up around his neck. He looked like a little boy.

"Mam always said that Thursdays were purple but we did at least agree that Saturdays were red."

"SHIT!"

From the back of the car, Dad suddenly burst into voice.

"What? What?"

"I forgot my meds. Shhhit."

"It's ok. We can get some more in the hospital. We'll be there in a minute."

I could see Dad getting worried in the back of the car. He'd started chewing the inside of his mouth and twiddling his fingers.

"Just take it easy driving." said Mum, placing her hand on my knee. "He doesn't like bumps."

The rest of the journey into hospital was slow and quiet. Dad, realising he had no anti-sickness medication on him, started burping. My finger was poised on the indicator ready to pull over should we need to.

When we got to the hospital, Mum and Dad

went ahead to get the radiotherapy done. I had a few business calls to make and I wandered in ten minutes later to find Mum sat in the waiting room, reading a copy of Bella. She had one leg crossed over the other and her reading glasses perched precariously on the end of her nose.

"Why does that telly have to be so loud?" she asked as I took my seat.

I looked up at the large flat screen that was screwed to the wall. David Dickinson's leather face was looking concerned as a fat lady quibbled over a couple of pounds for her shit statue of a cat. Meanwhile, in a nearby room, Dad was being screwed into his radiotherapy machine.

Ten minutes later, Dad emerged and we plonked ourselves back into the car and headed back to my house for a cuppa before he had to go back into hospital for his last overnight stay.

Clare bustled about busily but Dad sat quietly on the far end of the settee near the door. He didn't say a word.

"Cup of tea?" she asked.

"He's ok thanks." said Mum. "He's feeling a bit tender."

"Biscuit?" asked Clare. Dad shook his head. Clare gently tossed him the TV remote. She was trying to make him as comfortable as possible.

"Put on whatever you want." she said. David Dickinson soon disappeared, only to be replaced by a shiny fat man on Come Dine With Me. The fat man didn't even speak. He simply opened his mouth and let out large gutteral belch that shook his wet lips and quivered the sides of his fat, sweaty neck.

"Eurgh!" cried Dad, reaching for anything that could catch his sick. He leaned far forward but caught it in time.

"The dirty fat bastard!" he said, wiping his lips. "Fancy being proud of that."

Half an hour later and we were checking into his room at the hospital.

"En-suite?" said Mum, looking around. "Posh."

"They said last time that if I was good, I'd have an en-suite room."

A nurse came in with a fresh jug of water and placed it on his bedside table.

"Oo. Here again?" she squeaked.

"For one night only." said Dad. The nurse left and was quickly replaced by his nutritionist. A small North Walian, she began questioning Dad about what he'd drunk, what he'd eaten and what he'd shat out.

"Have you been taking your supplements?"

"I've had two today."

"How many did you have yesterday?"

"Erm. Two."

"You should really be taking five a day you know. I'll fetch you some more. Any particular flavours you like?"

"Fruits of the Forest please."

"If you don't drink them, we'll have to pump feed you."

Dad's face filled with fear.

"I'll have another two today and I'll have five tomorrow. I promise."

The nurse left us. Mum looked over the top of her glasses.

"Did you just lie to her?" she asked.

"What do you mean?" replied Dad.

"I've only seen you have one today."

"I had one when you went out." There was a brief silence in the room while we all judged the truth in his statement.

"They'll have to pump..."

"I HAD ONE WHEN YOU WERE OUT!"

"Alright! I was just saying that if you don't, you'll have to be pump..."

The word 'pump' seemed to make Dad jolt like he'd been poked with some kind of cattle prod.

"They are NOT pump-feeding me!"

"It's not a pump."

"I'M NOT HAVING IT!"

"If you let me finish what I'm trying to say, it's not a PUMP, it's a drip feed. You won't even notice it."

"I'll be drinking them. And that's that!"

Dad had taken his anti-sickness tablets and now lay on the bed, arms behind his head. Point made, I could tell he was glad just to be in one place where he could stretch out.

We left him there when visiting time was over. Hopefully this was his last overnight stay in hospital.

The next day, we picked him up and brought him and his Fruits of the Forest home. With the coal fire lit in the living room, Dad curled up on his settee and fell straight asleep.

******November 2002******

Me>Dad Guess where I am
Dad>Me Dunno
Me>Dad Weston-super-Mare seafront
Dad>Me What you doing there?
Me>Dad Sat in my car. Just having some lunch. It's pissing down here and out

*over the sea. **But I'm looking right over
the Bristol Channel and just wanted you
to know that I can see Barry bathed in
sunlight.***
***Dad>Me** That's because I'm here.*
***Me>Dad** God always shines his light on
you does he?*
***Dad>Me** Not at all. That's the sun shining
out of my arse x*

******

Tuesday 2nd October 2012

Dad had entered his final week of radiotherapy. He
had phoned me the previous Friday to let me know
that his consultant was pleased with his progress.
"He said that I was doing remarkably well." he kept
telling me "That's good isn't it?"

He only had four more planned visits to
the hospital and as I lay in bed that night, I was
convinced that Dad was going to go all the way and
drive himself to and from hospital right up until
the end of his treatment. He'd done himself proud.
But then my phone buzzed on my bedside table. It
was Mum.

Mum>Me Sorry it's short notice but can you
do the lifts for the rest of the week please?
Dad can't take any more x
Me>Mum Yeah, course. See you in the
morning xx

So far, we'd had a pretty good run of things. But the
last few days of his treatment were set to challenge
us all - and push Mum and Dad's relationship to

breaking point.

19 TINNED TANGERINES AND PEACH BLANCMANGE

Friday 5th October 2012

We'd all been on auto-pilot for the last few weeks with our visits to the hospital. Tiredness was drowning us all, forcing our worries to a dark corner at the back of our minds. But as the final week of treatment came looming over the horizon, the emotions we'd been experiencing at the start of the process were now beginning to trickle back. The tide was coming back in.

We were heading into hospital at 20mph. "Be careful going over bumps and no sudden jolts." were Mum's words to me as we had got into the car. I was under strict instructions not to burp. Food of any description was also not to be mentioned in any way, shape or form. My brother Dylan had been under the same rules the previous night but had still messed up by talking about his greasy jumbo sausage and chips. Dad had hurled up just a little of the food that he had left in his stomach. Dylan was very apologetic.

Driving so slowly was attracting the attention of drivers around us. Quickly filling my rear view mirror was some jumped up lad, all false tan and sunglasses, driving a yellow Mini. He looked about 12. Worst of all, he had a personalised number plate, which soon disappeared from view as he pushed his front grille close to my exhaust. He was swerving all over the road, trying to get around us. He pissed me off so much that I dropped down a gear just to watch him squirm and curse.

Mum was in the back of the car, on the phone, telling my sister how she'd been cleaning the house and tending to the garden. Dad was explaining to me in the best voice he could muster that he wasn't wanting visitors.

"I'm not being anti-social. I just don't want people around. I'm feeling very self-conscious and it's hard when the grandkids just stand there staring at me." he said. "I feel like some kind of freak show."

"THEY'RE NOT COMING!" said Mum from the back of the car, covering her phone mouthpiece with her hand. "HOW MANY MORE TIMES ARE YOU GOING TO GO ON ABOUT IT?"

"I was just explaining to..."

"Yes, but no-one is coming now please stop going on about it!" Mum sighed and took her hand away from the phone. "Sorry. Carry on." she said to my sister.

There was an awkward silence in the car, broken only by the tinny exhaust of the yellow Mini that finally overtook us.

"He was just telling me how he was feeling." I muttered. I felt I had to defend him in some small way. And Mum wasn't being nasty. Her patience was running out. Dad suddenly turned the conversation around.

"Every time I feel sick, I think of tangerines, those ones you get in a tin, served with peach blancmange. Mm. Biting into them and feeling them explode in your mouth. Lush." said Dad. I smiled, not knowing whether to return a comment about food or not.

We passed the park that we'd sat in on our

first day at the hospital.

"Seems like yesterday we were sat there eating our sandwiches." I said. My mind drifted back to that July day as we were sat there in the traffic. The last few months of summer seemed to have fluttered away in the ragged autumn winds.

Dad was kept waiting for a while before he finally headed in for his penultimate blast of radiotherapy. Mum was thumbing through a battered copy of Good Housekeeping and had stopped on a gardening feature when he was called in. She slid her reading glasses down from the top of her head, right to the end of her nose.

"I want mine just like this." she said, pointing to a picture in the magazine. "All trellising and plants." She was already planning her spring garden. In her mind, she was looking past Dad's illness and looking forward to daisy-fresh spring days full of clean laundry and open doors.

Dad finally emerged from the room and headed over to us.

"Bloods next." he said, throwing on his duffle coat.

The waiting room was like a giant ant colony with workers and patients scuttling round and bumping into each other. I don't think I'd ever seen it so busy. I pointed Dad to a seat in between two old women who sat hunched over like two grey gargoyles. But I had to stand.

Opposite me, leaning on his walking stick was a tall, elderly gentleman. He was dressed like some kind of farmer - a tweed jacket, a chequered shirt, a flat cap and a pair of grey trousers that were held up by a plastic-looking white belt. His deep-set eyes roamed slowly around the room.

"Tom Farley!" called one of the nurses,

appearing from the room. "Tom Farley?....No?"

A small puffy-faced man suddenly jumped up from his seat and quickly skulked into the room, clearly trying to avoid the angry little gargoyles who sat there huffing and snarling at everyone entering the bloods room. The farmer man lowered himself slowly into the now vacant seat and sighed. He was clearly in pain.

A female nurse stepped out from the room holding a clipboard.

"Emily Webley! Emily Webley!" she called out.

From around the corner waddled a larger lady. She seemed out of breath but made her way into the room.

Then there came a sudden squeak from the woman perched next to Dad.

"Excuse me! We've been here twenty minutes now! There are people turning up and going in ahead of us! I think it's disgusting! First 'im in there and then Wibbly Wobbly Webbly turns up and walks straight in!" she shrieked. Her voice was so high and shrill, it tickled my ear drums. The room hushed to listen to her screeching.

The nurse, big girl with heavy mascara, looked taken aback. We were all a bit alarmed.

"We're doing the best that we can. I'm sorry." she said.

"Well it's not good enough. This place is a disgrace!" squawked the woman again.

"Excuse me." said the nurse, taking a firm stance. "These are people who have just had a kidney test and have to have hourly bloods. YOU WILL BE SEEN TO BUT WHEN YOUR NAME IS CALLED!" She turned on her crocs and disappeared into the room, slamming the door hard behind her.

"I think it's disgusting!" muttered the woman again, hoping to gain the support of those sat around her. Dad just looked at me forlornly. This must have been the usual routine. I could tell that he just wanted to get home now.

"Robert Reeves!" Names were now ricocheting around the room. But not Dad's. I was shuffling from foot to foot, trying to stave off the dull pains growing in my heels. It was another forty minutes before Dad got called in, but Mum had already called me to ask for help carrying two large bags of medication.

The pharmacy was at the other end of the hospital. Mum and I were handed two heavy bags and a list of instructions. The bags included the supplements that Dad was supposed to be having five a day of, plus some anti-biotics for an infection he'd picked up.

"Are you coping?" I asked Mum as we made our way back to Dad.

"Just about. He keeps shouting at me."

"What for?"

"Because I keep asking him if he's taken his meds."

I sighed. Mum was only trying her best.

"I'm doing it to keep him alive and all he does is shout at me."

"Is he taking his medications?"

"I don't know. He says he is."

"I'm sure he feels like shit. He doesn't mean to shout. He's just frustrated at feeling so poorly all the time."

"I know that. But it still hurts. The annoying part about it is that I just want to jump in his face, poke my tongue out at him and say 'I told you that you should have gone to the doctor years ago instead of pretending that it was all ok.' But of course, I can't say that. I just have to bite my tongue. And on top of that, I'm lonely."

I felt a surge of love for my Mum. I put my arm tight around her and gave her a squeeze.

"Shall we have a day out next week? Just me and you?"

"Yeah. That'd be nice."

I kissed her on the top of her head before we tracked our way back to the busy waiting room.

Dad didn't speak as we left the hospital, apart from telling us about an old couple he'd sat next to the previous day. They were both in their eighties, he said - the man the one who was undergoing daily radiotherapy. They had a daughter who lived in England somewhere with her husband and young children. But they didn't want her to know about his illness. "She'd only worry." they said. So every day, they'd take drive the 200 mile round trip to the only place in Wales where they could get treatment.

The things you keep from loved ones to protect them from worrying.

I had to pull in at Danielle's house on the way home to pick up some things I'd left there. No sooner had I picked up my stuff than Mum was banging on the front door furiously.

I flung the door open. "What's happened?"

"You going to be long?"

"No. I'm coming now. Why? What's happened?"

"Nothing."

I pulled the door behind me and was surprised to find Dad stood outside of the car and flicking through some goodwill text messages on his phone. Mum quickly dived into the car while I loaded my stuff into the boot.

"What's happened?" I asked Dad.

"I can't sit in there with her. I can't."

"What are you on about?"

"She keeps nagging me, on and on. She wants me to take my medicines but I'm not taking them in the car. I'm not. She can wait until we get home."

It was a tense drive home and Dad headed straight for the settee where he crashed out straight away. The cat, happy to see him, bounced on over, but she was quickly swatted away. Dad was in no mood for anyone.

Mum got Dad comfy, lighting the coal fire and getting him a blanket before we drove out to pick up some shopping. With Mum not able to drive, and Dad too ill to, she needed to stock up. She bought him his tinned tangerines and his peach blancmange.

By the time I got home at teatime, I was completely exhausted. I closed my bedroom curtains, lay on my bed and closed my eyes.

"One more day. One more day." I kept repeating to myself as my body started twitching and jolting, falling into a deep sleep. I wouldn't see them now until Monday, the last planned day of his radiotherapy.

******Christmas 2012******

Hidden away in the middle of the Blue Anchor Inn sat my father. He had a big smile splashed across his face and his cheeks seemed to glow the same colour as the red lights on the Christmas tree behind him. I think it was down to the local ale he'd been supping or possibly the spicy parsnip soup he'd just devoured. It could have been the log fire that sizzled in the corner of the room. Either way, he was flanked on either side by his beloved family. He was finally happy.

And for once, I wasn't driving. I'd been able to savour the bleakness of the fields that once blazed in the summer months as we had made our way to the inn on the coast. Down on the hillsides, thin wisps of grey smoke spiralled up from the farmhouse chimneys. Lights on in their kitchens suggested that some Christmas baking was being prepared - perhaps some cakes or sausage rolls.

Our large table was strewn with empty soup bowls, scrunched up wrapping paper and gold tinsel. There was food, drink and laughter.

I turned to the bar, where my brother Dan was stood.

"Dan? Do you want to bring it over?" I called over to him.

A few minutes later, Dan was back at our table with a large silver platter. On it was a large bottle of champagne and a small collection of champagne flutes.

"Let's paaaaaaaaaaartay!" he shouted, announcing his arrival.

We all squealed as Dad popped off the cork from the champagne and he filled all our glasses.

"You haven't got loads each!" he said. It reminded me of the days as kids when we'd get cherryade from the Pop Man at Christmas. Dad would always serve up to make sure that no-one had more than anyone else.

I rose to my feet with my glass. I looked at Dad and smiled. After all he'd come through, it was so good to see him back to his usual self. I was beaming with pride.

"I'd like to raise a toast to Dad. For getting through a horrific year. I'd also like to raise a toast to Mum, for being there every step of the way. And I'd also like to raise a toast to us all for doing our best. It's been tough on all of us, but we're finally here. So here's to finally getting that all-clear, here's to a wonderful Christmas and to a better year in 2013..."

Our glasses pinged as we all toasted our wonderful Dad.

Bzzzzz. Bzzzz.

For a few seconds, I didn't know where I was or what was going on but it certainly wasn't Christmas. My bedroom had turned dark and cold as I had dozed. The incessant buzzing was my phone ringing, I knew that much. I flapped my hand around the bed, reaching out for it. I hated being woken.

"Hello?" I said groggily.

"Hi. It's me, Mum."

"Hiya. You ok?"

"No. I've just had the hospital on the phone."

"Oh no."

20 A SUMMER LONG GONE

Monday 8th October 2012

If Dad needed a kick up the arse to start taking his meds, it would be from a hospital telephone call.

Dad was pretending to relax on the settee, but he had one eye half open. He was listening.

Mum put the phone receiver down.

"Your kidney results are back. If you don't start drinking more, they'll be keeping you on a drip in A&E on Monday."

Dad sighed. I think he knew he hadn't been drinking enough. He'd been caught out.

"They'll be putting you on a pump." she said, leaving the living room so Dad could savour that thought.

***

The following Monday, it was Dad's final planned radiotherapy treatment. With the end now clearly in sight, we just wanted it over with.

I arrived to pick them up but I was slightly taken aback by the way Dad looked. He was stood there waiting in his duffle coat, looking sad. But his face was gaunt and white, apart from the red rawness down the side his neck that was creeping onto his face. Six weeks of radiotherapy does that to you.

Fortunately, Dad had pulled things back on the drinking front and he told us that he was not required to stay in when he sloped out of his review at the hospital. They were pleased with how he had handled things. There'd be a few more reviews to attend over the next few weeks but for now, it was one final blast of laser treatment.

Dad emerged from his radiotherapy with a wry smile on his face. In the back of my mind, I had been expecting a small brass band to pop up in the corner of the waiting room and deliver us a flourish of a fanfare as we left the building. But there was no brass band. There was no fanfare. We just left as we always had done.

It was an uneventful journey home apart from the sunbeams that grazed their long silvery arms along the coast as we arrived home. The coal fire was lit and Dad as usual, got straight onto the settee to rest. He'd done it. Mum disappeared down the hallway to put the kettle on.

"Time to rest." I said. "Well done. I'm proud of you."

"Thanks. And thanks for the last few months. You've been a rock and it would have been a lot more difficult without you."

"That's ok." I said. I picked up my car keys. "Get some sleep."

"Will do." said Dad, closing his eyes. "Love you."

I'd half-stepped out of the door when he said it.

"Pardon?"

"Love you." he said.

I couldn't help but raise the corner of my mouth. It was the first time he'd ever said it face-to-face. I stood there for a few moments, smiling to myself.

"Love you too Dad." I said. But I don't think he heard me. He was already fast asleep.

I fell into the car, closed the door and just sat there for a few minutes. I cast my mind back over the last few months. To the start of it all. That rainy day that I had that phone call. That tiny office we'd all sat in. Andy Murray. Loudmouth Jim. I wondered where he was now. I wondered if he was still sat in that hospital bed simmering like a volcano about to erupt. I thought about our visit to the café in the park. I thought about the guy who had been stood reading the thank you cards on the wall of the hospital. I wondered if he was still there, or whether there was a thank you card on the wall from his family to the staff. I thought about our local cinema, now being rebuilt as some fancy flats for pensioners. I thought about Thomas and his cowboy hat, probably now long-discarded. I thought about Lucy. I wondered where she was. I thought about my little furry friend who we'd left at our old house. I thought about the tinned tangerines and the peach blancmange. I thought about the rain. And I thought about what I did next.

'Go home and have a cup of tea.' I thought to myself. I started the car and put the heaters on.

Then I headed back to my life as I'd left it back in June.

******

EPILOGUE

August 2013

Dad was given the all-clear for this throat cancer in April 2013. Sadly, a few weeks later, during a scan in preparation for some post-treatment trials, cancer was found in his lung. He had half his lung removed but later tests showed that the cancer had spread to his spine and liver, and remained in his lung.

He fought the disease vigourously, but when told that they were considering withdrawing his chemo, he resigned himself to his fate.

August 9th 2013

Last night, I held the hand of my dying father. Dad had beautifully soft hands, despite the years of hard slog and night shifts he'd put in while we slept as children. And as dusk fell outside, and as the drizzle pattered on the hospital windows, we both drifted into some kind of place. For me, we weren't hidden away in a dark hospital room full of tubes and strange noises – we were holding hands and heading to the local park for a kickabout with a rugby ball on one of those endlessly sunny Saturday afternoons.

Dad always taught us to always look at the positive side of things, whatever we were faced with. His illness crippled him, but it also brought us together as a family. He never moaned. He taught us how to believe and fight for the things we love. He raged against the dying of the light, boy did he rage. And I love him for that. But he waited until no-one was looking to steal away into the night and join the family who were waiting for him. He didn't want any of us to have the memories of him leaving us.

The disease took his body, but it can never take away the love and the memories of a great man. I am, and will always will be, proud to say that this was my dad.

ABOUT THE AUTHOR

Patric is an award-winning writer and author based in Cardiff, Wales.

A former English teacher, Patric has been working as a freelance writer since 2005. He has had work published in the Western Mail, South Wales Echo, Wales on Sunday, The Guardian, WM magazine, Your Wedding, OneWales, Americymru and RedHanded magazine.

In 2007, Patric and his business partner, Danielle, set up Rhiwbina Living magazine in Cardiff to help promote local business. By popular demand, a second magazine, Whitchurch and Llandaff Living was launched in 2008. Both magazines have gained critical acclaim, and was recognised by The Guardian as a '...vital source of news in the community'.

In 2012, Patric scooped the 'Best Writing on a Blog' Award at the 2012 Wales Blog Awards for his blog, Do Not Go Gently. He is a current contributor to the Huffington Post.

You can find more at www.patricmorgan.co.uk

5981480R00067

Printed in Great Britain
by Amazon.co.uk, Ltd.,
Marston Gate.